WHY

WHY

Sexual Abuse and Pornography:
*Daily Battles That Can Cause a
Lifetime of War*

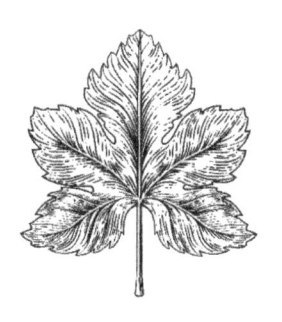

Carmen Watt

© 2021 Carmen Watt

The text from this book may be quoted in any form (written, visual, electronic, or audio), without written permission from the publisher, provided that the text quoted does not amount to more than 20 percent of the total text of the work in which they are quoted. When quoted, the following credit lines must appear on the copyright page of the work:

"Quotations are from Why®. Copyright © 2021 by Carmen Watt. Used by permission. All rights reserved."

Quotations in excess of these guidelines must be approved in writing by Carmen Watt.

Requests should be submitted to Carmen Watt.

carmen@watt-group.com

Unless otherwise noted all scriptures taken from the New King James Version®. Copyright

© 1982 by Thomas Nelson. Used by permission. All rights reserved.
Scripture quotations marked (NLT) are from the Holy Bible, New Living Translation®. Copyright © 1996 by Tyndale House Publishers, Inc. Used by permission. All rights reserved.

Scripture quotations marked (NIV) are taken from the Holy Bible, New International Version®, NIV®. Copyright © 1973, 1978, 1984, 2011 by Biblica, Inc.™ Used by permission of Zondervan. All rights reserved worldwide. www.zondervan.com The "NIV" and "New International Version" are trademarks registered in the United States Patent and Trademark Office by Biblica, Inc.™

ISBN: 978-1-7379297-0-3

DEDICATION

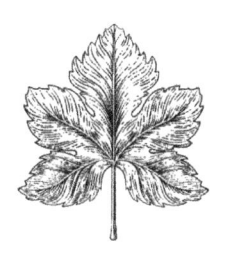

To my lovely husband, Wessel
and my precious children,
Keenan, Ciara, Camren, and Elijah.

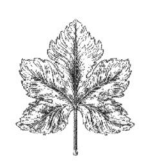

CONTENTS

Acknowledgements 1

Foreword 3

Introduction 7

Chapter 1: Arriving In Egypt 10

Chapter 2: Chains Of Bondage 17

Chapter 3: A Slave Between The Pyramids 31

Chapter 4: Fleeing From Egypt 50

Chapter 5: Standing In Front Of The Red Sea 59

Chapter 6: Crossing Over 65

Chapter 7: Stepping Into The Dessert 79

Chapter 8: Trust, Denial And Failure In The Wilderness .. 94

Chapter 9: Stuck With Egypt's Diseases And
My Manna 104

Chapter 10: The Law And Love 120

Chapter 11: Golden Calves And Pornography 133

Chapter 12: Wandering To Canaan 142

Chapter 13: Running Out Of Time 149

Chapter 14: Death In The Wilderness 155

Chapter 15: Entering Canaan... 162

Chapter 16: The Grapes And The Giants 168

Suggested Readings And Resources 175

Biography.. 178

End Notes 180

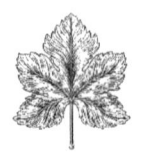

ACKNOWLEDGEMENTS

Where does one begin to say thank you? What words can truly share my appreciation? I must start with you, my reader. Thank you for walking with me on my journey to Canaan, for carrying my story with you and for your precious time. This book is written for you. This book is written for you and for every child that experienced loss, pain and suffering because of sexual abuse.

Thank you, Brandi, my editor and writing coach, for believing in me and my story, which is no different from the Israelites' story and many people all over the globe. Thank you for taking my hand on this unknown writing journey. You empowered me.

Thank you to my four wonderful children – Keenan, Ciara, Camren, and Elijah. You inspire me daily and I cannot think of a life without you four Watt's. Thank you for your endless support, and "you can do it, Mom" encouragements when I wanted to give up. This book is written for you.

Thank you to my wonderful husband, Wessel. Thank you for believing in me and thank you for giving me wings when I thought I would never fly. I never thought such a broken, mixed-up kid like me could ever be loved and accepted. But you proved me wrong, every time you chose me. Your life has proven that this book has the power to break any chains, to restore people completely and find true freedom. I will forever be grateful for the power of these words on these pages because this book has caused us to love unconditionally, forgive without blame and to live more authentically. We will never be the same again. Thank you for being the most amazing life partner and the truest of friends.

And finally, to the friend like no other, Jesus. My Savior. The King of the World. Thank you for your endless mercy and grace. Thank you for your Spirit that uplifted me in my darkest days and your counsel that upheld me when I saw no way out. Thank you for pruning me and showing me how much you truly love me. Thank you that you showed me what real love is. Thank you for making me strong in you and thank you for turning my nightmares in to beautiful dreams.

Cheers to the next 40 years with you, Jesus.

FOREWORD

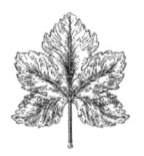

Wow! It has been an 18-year long rollercoaster ride! Expectant, fast, exciting, unpredictable, exhilarating, sometimes uphill and you bet, scary at times. Having met Carmen more than twenty years ago and spending the past almost eighteen years together as husband and wife, and raising four kids together, has been great, but tough. I think we are probably two of the sharpest blades around, that is if you believe in the saying: "Iron sharpens iron."

Carmen has always been on a journey of gaining knowledge and a deeper understanding of how people behave and what influences them. Together we have tried on numerous occasions to try and puzzle out exactly what causes certain behavior and how to rectify, improve, change, and grow in our own lives… only to realize after some alterations in behavior, still more work and change is needed. Some issues are just under the surface and easy to identify and rectify – almost common.

But it is those much deeper, darker secrets that we bury and try to hide far, far away that can cause a lifetime of sorrow and pain.

I came back from a 2-week fishing trip in New Zealand and was handed a 40-page booklet by Carmen. While I was out fishing, she felt the need to pen down her past and the horrific things that happened in her life. Some of the events we have discussed while doing life together, but never in such detail. The 40-page booklet has evolved into the book that you hold in your hands today. I have read this book numerous times and can't believe how blind I was to trauma and the effect it has on human behavior. The potential for shackling, numbing, de-activating, eliminating a full and healthy life, I was ignorant of, for sure. I had a different upbringing with less trauma and was uneducated to the existence and effects of trauma. Trying to do life together in an ever-changing environment coupled with the aftereffects of trauma was incredibly challenging. By reading **Why,** I got a much clearer picture of trauma, its effects and how to identify it sooner. Also, I learned what to do and what not to do. Not all trauma events are the same, but they all influence our perceptions, thinking and behavior.

Since the first writings, we have spent many times discussing the events of the past and how it has shaped us, and also how it has robbed us from a more fulfilled and happy life. If only it was possible to deal with the past sooner. But we did not know how, and we both entered our relationship with the undealt baggage of the past: the pain, the shame, the guilt, and the walls we had built to protect us. Because we are unable to see what other people are thinking and what scenes are playing out in their brains – the memory flashes, their thoughts, the recalled traumatic events – it is crucial for all of us to be able to collectively deal with these in the lives of people who we love and care for. It is incredibly important that we take note of the state of our souls and ensure that just as we work at attaining a healthy body and spiritual life, we also do our best in restoring our souls.

This book will give you more insight on the "realness" of trauma, as well as the effects of sex, pornography, and child-abuse – be it sexual, verbal or physical. It has enabled me to speak more openly about events in my own life, as well as to have more empathy with my fellow human beings. Reading Carmen's story and the torture she had gone through, long after the events, has arrested my heart and challenged me regarding the secrets I kept and the way I behaved. **Why**, allowed me to compare my life's events with not only her life but also with those of the Israelites during their 40-year journey through the desert on the way to Canaan. I was confronted with my own mistakes and ill behavior, and I was able to start a road of openness and recovery that I have never known before.

It is a journey that I am on, that while I don't know the end destination, I know that I am free, walking in the light, with no past events and mistakes haunting me anymore. It is a journey that I want to keep staying on and take others with me to also experience a life lived in the open – a real and free life!

Wessel Watt, *Carmen's Husband*

INTRODUCTION

It overwhelms me when I think about you holding this book in your hand. Firstly, it is crazy to imagine that someone would take time to read something so real and raw like my story. And secondly, I am secretly childlike in my excitement for you to find "truth-bombs" hidden by God all through these pages. I might not be the best writer, but in Him, I sure had the best co-writer with me.

I experienced the power of healing with every word I misspelled, every grammar mistake I made and every uncertainty I felt. I started off by tripping over my words, to ending with you on my mind. If only you find one truth of God's love in this book, every teardrop that I spilled was worth it. I guess my story is like many children that have gone through child abuse, but I want to believe that it is different. It is different because I found freedom after years of pain and grief.

You will find real life experiences in these pages, some of them were just me sharing my heart authentically. Maybe you'll see yourself in some of them. Perhaps it will bring relief to you to know that you are not alone. The aftermath of sexual abuse is real and the scars of it deep. Freedom looks impossible from the receiving end of abuse but remember the "truth-bombs" I told you about. You will surely find them while you scroll through these pages.

I had to get some help in unpacking this whole journey of mine to freedom and I could not think of better writing partners than the Israelites. I often saw them in my own narrative and in doing so, did not feel so insecure about my own life. They really were a bunch of stubborn and disoriented people. Maybe they too struggled with their identity. But God never blamed them for behaving like slaves while being free. He patiently and consistently drew them closer to His heart.

In every chapter of this book you are holding, God weaved in his desire for us to be free. That is why I share with a true and vulnerable heart. He wants you to see that He never gives up on you, never. He never gave up on the Israelites. Was the journey in the Wilderness difficult? You bet! But nothing stopped God from pursuing them. Nothing stopped God from pursuing me.

My wish for you is to meet the God of Israel between these pages. But my ultimate hope would be for you to give Jesus a chance to show you the way to freedom.

He is a true friend, trust me.

WHY

CHAPTER 1

Arriving in Egypt

"Children are the hands by which we take hold of heaven."[1]

Henry Ward Beecher

I was a joyful little girl once. Sexual abuse and exposure to pornography at a very young age made my life a nightmare and many days I wished to disappear and never breath another breath of air. I remember my helplessness and confusion. The gripping torment of that pain haunted me. For many years. I had not always been sad, helpless, and scared. I had not always been filled with buckets of anxiety and pain. I was once *normal*.

I was born in 1980 in beautiful sunny South Africa. The rainbow nation of the world. I was born 40 years ago during the time of apartheid. While I was writing this book, it seems like the whole world is part of apartheid. COVID-19 hit the world in 2020 and now somehow in some way or other, we were all apart. More distant and divided than ever before. Social distancing, staying at home and being separated from one another is the life we all had to get used to. This is only a small glimpse of what apartheid was like. We as people are being separated from one another not able to connect as we used to. We are forced not to touch one another, to distance ourselves from one another and even staying away from family members is our new *apartheid*. Unfortunately, *apartheid*, sickness, corruption, racism, hate, and pain are still evident all over our world and seem impossible to escape from.

I was not aware of the challenges during apartheid, I was too young, and I did not grow up with racist or prejudice parents. There was no talking about any culture or race in any negative or bias way in our home. I just remember that we lived somewhat apart from each other. Black people and white people were separated. We were separated by our color and culture. We did not "mingle" and do everyday things together like going to school, visiting restaurants, or sharing a public park. That was "normal." I knew when I looked around, I did not see a lot of black people hanging around our house, visiting or coming over for dinner. That was not allowed. I did not ask any questions. **Why** would you if that is what you know to be normal.

I'm a real 80's girl and I still listen to *Roxette* on full blast and luckily my ears have had no dramatic degeneration over the years. I am the third child of four and, yes, you can call me a middle child, but that would put a certain label on me. *I do not like labels.* I was always called "sensitive" from a very young age. For some reason I never liked it if someone said: "You're so sensitive." It sounded very offensive, pathetic, and lame, it never sounded like a compliment, especially when it was portrayed as a negative character trait and that it would be best for you to change that. *I never got to that.*

While growing up I always lived with this feeling of being left out, I struggled to fit in and could never reach that feeling of belonging, a feeling of acceptance by people. Not even in my own family, and I never understood **why**. I had a wonderful family and like most children did not need much growing up. At that stage in your life, your family is all you have and the center of your being. It is your people, your tribe, and your haven. As a young child you have this inherent need to belong and to be accepted in your tribe. We as humans are made that way. You want to know that when you are not there anymore, that your chair is empty, your voice is missed, and that you most definitely are irreplaceable. Belonging is one of our core human needs. I'm sure you will agree.

I grew up knowing that family is important. Family is your people; the people that would be the closest to you your whole life. I was told that family is everything. I grew up with a family that loved food and the fellowship that food created, like many other families too. That fellowship around the table created small moments of belonging and cohesiveness and then it also created moments of utter devastation. Food plays such a big role in the lives of families and their culture. The time spend around the dinner table is where memories are made... Or nightmares.

In my second year of Primary school, we moved to another house. My dad had a magical touch when it came to houses. He is a restorer of note. He would buy a house, we would move in, and after all the magic happened, he would sell it and we had to move to a new home. (Nowadays it is called house flipping.) I had to change schools and struggled to adjust to my new environment. Looking back, I knew that that was the first of many traumatic experiences for me. *Change.* I struggled with change just like most children do, especially when your safety was threatened. When you are young, it is very difficult to communicate what you feel and what you need at every given time. Communication for a small child is still a learning process. And from experience, I know that play is mostly how children communicate to the world. They often do not have the vocabulary to express themselves in a way that an adult would. Children should be taught how to communicate their emotions and feelings preferably in a safe environment. If they do not have the skills and abilities to do that, they will easily camouflage their fears, hurt, and pain. When you do not see their pain, it does not mean that it is not there. When they do not verbalize their fear, it does not mean it does not exist. But when you look closely at children's behavior you will be able to see. I guess it is normal for 8-year-old's to still find their special place in a family and in the world, it takes time to develop and find your own unique identity, an identity that we all strive for. One that makes sense to us and one that is acceptable to the world. One that screams: *"Hey world, this is me."* And be proud of that *me*. And love that *me*. Luckily, I always had a remedy for feeling alone and confused, my music.

I can still feel the trembling vibrations of my new CD player on full blast listening to "Another One Bites the Dust" by Queen. I listened to music for all the reasons people listen to music and I probably had a few of my own dark reasons. I listened to music to relax, to party, to dance, to cry, to mourn, to numb out, to disappear – the list was endless. My reason was mostly to be transported to another world, a different place, a place where I felt safe, shielded, and unseen. A place where no one knew my name. A place where I could be who I wanted to be. A place where no one told me what to do or how to do it. A place where I could choose which words enter my soul and which words should drown in their poison. A place where I had control over my eyes. A life where my body was my own. A space where I could dream, create, and build my own world. While my music played, I became someone else, if only for that short while. That short while was sometimes just enough. Enough to carry on. In the days where I decided to carry on my music was always close by. My music was never only for me to hear. I made pretty sure of that. I listened to music on full volume, wanting to make sure that it blocked out all other noises and voices that I might hear. Even my own inner voice was drowned by my ear-deafening music. My inner voice that daily screamed: *"What is wrong with you? What is wrong with you?"* Loud was never too loud for me. It was short squirts of moments in time where I could experience some relief and a few drops of happiness. My happiness was short-lived and scarce.

Music can play a very significant role in children's lives, especially in their formative years. It has the ability to save a child, to help him cope with what seems unbearable. Music can become a friend to many children. An invisible friend, but always there. It became my friend every single day.

Being part of a big family was a blessing and some days a curse. We always had one another and being around those you love made life beautiful and worth living. Even bleak days can turn into summery days when you have family and friends that loves you. Of course, like all families we had difficult times, every day was not perfect and yes there were a lot of fighting. That did not mean that we did not love each other. I often think of Joseph when I reflect on my own life. He was also part of a big family, but his siblings did not love him as much as my siblings loved me. Mine did not want to kill me. *Maybe some days they felt they wanted to.*

Joseph's siblings did get rid of him, and through all his trials and tribulations that you might have read in the Bible, he ended up in the house of the Pharaoh of Egypt.

Joseph was an amazing brother, and he did not plan revenge on his brothers for selling him. Instead, he saved them and blessed them. We definitely need more Josephs in families today. God appeared to Jacob, Joseph's father, during a time of great famine and told him not to be afraid to go to Egypt to ask for help, because He would be with him and eventually turn his small family into a great nation; then He would bring them back from Egypt and they would settle in the land of Canaan. (Sounds like a simple and easy plan, right?)

Joseph's family survived the famine that overtook the entire land. Joseph, the wonderful brother that he was, secured property for his family and they all moved to the northeastern Nile delta. There the Pharaoh gave Jacob and his family fertile land and the family which is now known as the Israelites grew from being only descendants, to a tribe of people that loved each other and stayed in Egypt with Joseph. It was initially a good exchange and a blessing for God's people; but unfortunately, that Pharoah died and those after him weren't as kindhearted.

In the meantime, that small Israelite family grew into a great people. I grew, too and we all know that *growing up is never easy.*

CHAPTER 2

Chains of Bondage

"Trauma has the ability to change the very essence of who you are."

Carmen Watt

I still love to watch as they send people off into space. I am not an American, but I can just imagine how exciting it must have been to be part of a country that did such groundbreaking work. The Hubble space station launch and deployment in April 1990 marked the most significant advance in astronomy since Galileo's telescope. I was ten. I remember it like it was yesterday. Oh, the adventure that awaited those astronauts! During this season of my life, I often felt that it would be better to be in space rather than to be on earth. I also wished to be an astronaut like most children, but my reasons had nothing to do with exploration. When you are "up there," nothing "down here" has any bearing on you. It would have been an excellent escape plan. Slowly, our family life had deteriorated, and I started to notice it more and more every day. When you are young, you do not see everything the way it really is. You experience things through your five senses and your gut. Small children are very aware of the atmosphere and the tension even if no words are spoken. Sometimes you are blindfolded; other times you have earplugs in. Sometimes you hear things that you wish you did not. But my visceral experiences told me something was wrong, and my eyes saw more and more of what was really going on. *I did not want to see it.*

There was constant conflict and strive between my father and mother. For some reason they could never get along. I am sure they did but the overwhelming fear surrounding the conflict made it so I could never see the other days when we all were just "a happy family." The "happy family" moments slowly happened less and less. My parents were literally petrol (or you might say gas) and fire. And those flames of strife and disunity easily jumped across to the children. Just like flames normally do. If you have ever seen wildfires, you know what I am talking about. I was constantly aware of the tension, the atmosphere, and the fear hovering in the air. The discord and ceaseless friction only increased. It would continue for days on end and then finally stopped, but only after a volcano of negative emotions erupted all over the house. When volcanos erupt, they do not always pre-warn people. Then we really experienced the heat of conflict and had to live with the remaining lava flow, tip toeing around every corner avoiding unnecessary burns.

Children should never fear their parents, but I did. And I know there are many more children that do. One thing I have learned to be true, is that young children should never try to be the fire extinguisher. It will always end up badly for them. You will walk away with second degree burns and will forever have the scars to remind you of that. Children cannot put out a fire between two parents; that is not their role as children. They are not supposed to protect their parents from one another. No child should be part of domestic violence in the first place. But somehow adults think children are immune to domestic violence. They think small children don't understand, they won't notice, but they do. Go look at the statistics, you will see the suffering of children between the numbers.

I saw the scars but still did not really understand what was going on. I could not put the puzzle pieces together. **Why** do they hate each other and **why** are we part of this love-hate relationship? **Why** did you have children? Is it my fault that you are fighting? Children ask these questions. **Why** did they marry in the first place? Is this what love is? A lot of children have these thoughts too. **Why** marry someone and then fight for years on end? They were a combination of two very different people trying to do life together and it just did not work for them.

My dad was and still is quite a genius, just a very scary genius. I loved my dad, I still do. But I was very fearful of my dad. I remember his anger explosions and I also remember his beautiful grey eyes and skewed smile when he was in a good mood. I loved that about him. He was a super strong-willed man, an absolute perfectionist with a heart of gold. He was also a very highly strung person, with extreme demands on his life. Only excellence was good enough for my dad. Nothing less. Stupidity or lack of understanding made him extremely angry. His impatience with ignorance, uneducated and dishonest people made him burst with frustration. He did not only live by very high standards, but he also expected those around him to meet those standards.

I would often hide in my room just to escape his presence. When I think back on those days, I do not know **why** I feared him. I feared the conflict that surrounded him and his relationship with my mother. One thing I still treasure until today is the love for music he shared with me. He had a deep passion for music and shared that almost every day for hours with us as his family. That is how I found my love for music. He would share this love for music with anyone who made time to sit, listen and be with him. He communicated through his music. I understood more of him, his life and his past by sharing his love for music. When tear drops ran down his cheeks, I knew he was feeling something that he was not able to explain and he was sharing that feeling with me, unintentionally. Many times, I could feel his pain while sitting next to him. No one would say a word, it was not necessary, the music spoke for us.

WHY

I loved my dad but was often torn between my dad being a very unstable person and my dad being the coolest, most fun person to be with. He was my dad. I loved him in any shape or form. Even if he was very harsh at times. I loved listening to his stories of his extremely poor upbringing, moving from Zimbabwe to South Africa at a very young age. He also struggled with *change* and found it very difficult to adapt to his new environment and his new home. He overcame all the odds and difficulties. He was an English-speaking boy that had to learn a new language and could not understand one word of Afrikaans. His family life was not easy, and his father struggled to make ends meet. I thought my dad was a hero. He survived many traumatic experiences in his life like many in his generation did. I always felt my father was carrying a burden regarding his children and his family life. I knew he carried a big responsibility for being the breadwinner and wanting to provide in abundance for his family. Looking back, I realized it was the destructive relationship they lived in. But I knew he loved his family very much. I believed he loved us as much as he possibly could but his relationship with my mother made it very hard. They both made it very difficult for each other. And for us.

Most of my young life I was torn between my parents. I did not know whose side to choose, because I loved both dearly. I struggled to get closer to my father because I feared him, and I wanted to protect my mother, but at the same time I needed to protect myself. My mother was this beautiful, feisty woman that did not back down. My dad must have known that he was marrying a woman that was also exposed to fire and had her own burn wounds while growing up in South Africa. She too had to try and overcome many events in her life that she struggled to speak about. But my mother had the same need as any other child in this world. To be loved unconditionally, to be safe, to be valued and to be accepted. I do not know if my dad ever met these needs, and I don't think one of them understood the root of their disunity.

It is necessary to treat the wounds of pain, rejection and hurt while you are young so that the scars do not show up in your adult life. Unfortunately, most of the wounds in children's lives do not heal by only putting on a few bandages. Sometimes, it needs surgery. It was not easy to experience this roller coaster of a relationship with two people you really love. There were days that I could not take it anymore. I could not stand the yelling, the swearing, the anger, and the discord between them. But hey, we were still this perfect and "happy" family.

Even in all this chaos, I still experienced blessings in my life as a child. My father was the best example of providing for a family I have ever experienced. I never lacked any material thing and was seen as a very privileged child compared to my friends. My dad sacrificed a lot and was always working hard towards leaving a legacy for us. He valued family. Unfortunately, it was not enough.

Viewer Discretion Advised

During the highs and lows of growing up there were also glimpses of hope. I experienced those glimpses when we were together as a family watching movies. My family loved movies. We had movie nights, movie mornings, movie afternoons. We were movie and music fanatics. We watched everything and the TV in our house was on 24 hours a day. My mother would get furious because my dad would let us watch movies that were inappropriate for our age. We were conservative, yet very liberal while growing up. Two extremes under one roof. My mother never won the movie battle.

We had wonderful values put in place but somehow there was no boundaries or rules when it came to that little sign on the cover of a movie. You know, those PG-13 or NC-17 signs? It was there for a reason; I am sure you will agree. They say it is true that the more you watch over-aged things, the more your mind adapts and later you become numb to violence and sex scenes. That which was disturbing to you once will not bother you anymore. It might be true for the rest of the world, but not for me. I was a *sensitive* viewer my whole life. What I watched impacted me on a large scale.

Research shows that "media has a tremendous capacity to teach. Excessive media use, particularly where the content is violent, gender-stereotyped, and/or sexually explicit, skews children's world view, increases high-risk behaviors, and alters their capacity for successful and sustained human relationships."2

My days were filled with movies and music and somewhere in the house there would always be something playing. I had free access to mostly anything with little to no boundaries and was not aware of any danger regarding movies. It was normal to me. I was innocent and naive. Like many other days I would watch TV or listen to music when I was bored, and it was one of those days that changed my life completely. This specific day turned out to be totally different than any other day. I was totally caught off guard and unprepared for what followed next. If I could go back to that day. I would. I would want to change what happened. I would change what was playing. I would change what I saw.

It was pornography.

I did not know what it was called then but I soon found out what it was. Two people naked, doing something that looked amazing. It immediately awakened my human curiosity and I thought that this is the most interesting thing I have ever seen. Unfortunately, though the pornography was found by an innocent child, I just had to watch it again. I could not stop watching it. My body responded in a way that I was not familiar with.

I was hooked.

What I saw must have been love. Physical affection was not something that I experienced much as a child and when I did, it was never enough for me. I guess you can never out-hug a child. I am a very affectionate person, and physical touch is something that I craved as a child. What I saw made me feel warm and fussy inside. It was as if I felt something for the first time, and what I felt was something that I had really missed. *I know, weird!* I wondered **why** I felt so good about it, **why** I felt so much comfort through watching it. But I am sure I knew I was not supposed to feel like this, and I was not supposed to watch it.

I think it was then and there that I was instantly enslaved. I was exposed to a thing that could mimic love, a counterfeit product of love. I understand it now, but I did not back then. How could I? In a way it made me feel safe. I felt safe while watching it. I was hungry to experience safety as a young girl. My dysfunctional habits started, and masturbation and pornography became part of my daily life. Silently, I escaped from the havoc in my family life to my new prison. I only realized that I was a slave when I could not think about anything else, but that. My thoughts were engulfed by all the images I saw. Day in and day out, my mind became bombarded with naked people.

> "It would be better for him if a millstone were hung around his neck, and he were thrown into the sea, than that he should offend one of these little ones."
>
> **Luke 17:2 NKJV**

I stumbled and had no one to pick me up. It was a big, big terrible accident. It was not supposed to have happened to me. I was a beautiful, young, innocent blond-haired girl that liked to play outside and do things that children love to do. **Why** did they do this to me? I immediately jumped to adulthood, and I skipped my developing phases that were very crucial to all my development areas, and those of any young child. From brain development to emotional development. My brain was not prepared to see so many naked people doing things that were not for my eyes to see. I was bound up with harsh chains in seconds. But I know I was not the only one. Today there are millions of children chained to pornography.

> *"Did you know that children and youth are more vulnerable to pornographic images than adults because of mirror neurons in the brain, which convince people that they are experiencing what they see? Mirror neurons play an important role in how children learn. Children learn in large part by imitation, with mirror neurons involved in the process of observing what other people do and imitating those behaviors. Pornography may have stronger effects among children and youth than any other form of media because it shows a much higher degree of sexual explicitness."*[3]

Trapped

Let us get back to where the Israelites find themselves. They grew to a wonderful, fruitful tribe but unfortunate they grew to a size that scared the Pharaoh.

Israel was from the beginning destined to be a blessed nation. Under a previous administration, the Israelites had royal permission to live in the land and to work it. But now that was all going to change. The new king of Egypt sensed in their numbers a threat to his nation, and he decided to change things. The Egyptians started to use force on the Israelites. The king had no compassion for the people of Israel and chose to forget all that Joseph had done for Egypt. He decided to act against the growing influence and numbers of Israel. He called his council together, and they advised him to enslave these people and oppress them before they grew too powerful.

Pharaoh started to limit the personal freedoms of the Israelites, put heavy taxes on them and recruited their men into forced labor under the supervision of harsh taskmasters. The children of Israel had to build cities, erect monuments, construct roads, work in the quarries, and make bricks and tiles. But the more the Egyptians oppressed them, and the harder the restrictions imposed upon them, the more the children of Israel increased and multiplied. Finally, when the Pharoah saw that forcing the Hebrews to do hard work failed in suppressing their rapidly growing numbers, he decreed that all the newly born male children of the Hebrews were to be thrown into the Nile River. *Pure evil, don't you think?* Only daughters were permitted to live. It is very interesting to see how threatened the Pharoah of Egypt was by the tribe of Israel. For years, it was prophesied that Israel would be a blessed nation governed by God.

My enemy was also threatened by my life from the day I was born. His plan was always to keep me away from my true identity and true freedom, he convinced me to believe that I would always be bound by pornography and sex with no way out. For many years there was no way out. I did not even smell freedom and there was no sign of freedom anytime soon.

I wondered how it must have felt to be Moses, have you thought about it? He was a Jew by birth and raised in an Egyptian palace. How did he manage those two different believe and value systems? *Now that is what you call living a double life!* Moses was exposed to two different upbringings for sure. He had exposure to two different believe systems and we all know how that turned out for him when he had to choose which Moses he wanted to be. The moment he killed that Egyptian taskmaster, when he defended one of his own, the choice was made. I was brought up very similar to Moses. Two types of upbringings competing with one another. In this wrestling with my two lives of who I am, I had loneliness that followed me everywhere.

Loneliness.

The pain from feeling alone. It is a deep pain of being forgotten, being misunderstood, being left out, excluded, and being exposed to things that were never my choice. *I felt isolated.* Fear became my shadow. My brain formed a path and through the years that path has been dug deeply into my mind. It did not leave much room for school and normal childlike things. I was an under performer, undiagnosed with dyslexia and as you will see in later chapters, ADD as well. I developed learning disabilities and could not concentrate or focus to finish any task. I had a damaged brain as the result of pornography and all the strive in my home. I cannot remember one thing I learned in school. Obviously, I did learn something, I just cannot remember any of it. *Trauma often creates memory loss.* From age 11 onwards there is not much that I remember. There was no space for any other thoughts in my mind except those images of the pornography I saw and the guilt I carried with it. Children must connect a positive emotion to a learning experience for it to last as a very important long-term memory. My positive memories were few. Other memories you wish you could forget. Only later in my life did I really get to understand what that trauma did to my brain. I guess my parents thought I was stupid and a under performer and they probably made peace with it. I was traumatized, badly and I never realized it. Nobody did. Not even my parents. I believe very few parents know that viewing pornography at a very young age is traumatizing to a small child. It is abusive and destructive. This very destructive behavior continued, and shame and guilt filled my mind every single day. I felt deprived, as if something had been stolen from me. I was very mad, mad at myself. This was all my fault. I wish I had never been placed in that position. I had to blame someone, and I could only blame myself. I did not want to be a *bad* child and blame my parents. So, I stuck with the fact that only myself was to blame. I was flawed mentally.

"Did you know that medical literature supports the premise that a person with one addiction is likely to have another? Youth are more likely than adults to be diagnosed with more than one mental health issue, including sexual acting out, substance abuse, and other disorders. Personality disorders, mood and anxiety disorders, and substance abuse and dependence are associated with sexual compulsivity. People recovering from drug addiction are at risk for sexual addiction, as they may "engage in substitute behaviors that serve similar pleasurable functions." Physical, sexual, family, and social trauma can also lead to the development of sexual addiction or compulsivity."[4]

My soul was ruined, and I made peace with the fact that I would always be a slave. I was no different to the Israelites. They too became somewhat content with the mistreatment of the hand of the hard Egyptian task masters, they made peace with their lives for 400 years.

Imagine that.

CHAPTER 3

A Slave Between the Pyramids

"Childhood abuse cast a shadow the length of a lifetime."[5]

Herbard Ward

When I think of a slave, my mind always drifts off to the life of Nelson Mandela. He served all together twenty-seven years in prison and was released in 1990. Mandela was part of official talks to end white minority rule and in 1991, he was elected ANC President to replace his friend, Oliver Tambo. In 1993, he and President F.W. de Klerk jointly won the Nobel Peace Prize and on April 27, 1994, he voted for the first time in his life. On May 10, 1994, he was inaugurated as South Africa's first democratically elected president. That was the end of apartheid. I was 14 years old.

I do not know what is worse: twenty-seven years in a 6 x 4-meter cell or four hundred years under the Egyptian rule? At least the Israelites had the reassurance that their stomachs would be full. I do not think Mandela could choose his dinner. *Four hundred* years is more than ten generations. I have always wondered **why** they did not try to escape. They did not once flee or fight back. I wonder if Mandela also studied the Exodus and if God's people also inspired him to write his book: *Long Walk to Freedom.* It was sure a long walk for him, as well. Mandela did not make peace with his circumstances. His freedom was offered many times under specific circumstances, but he never chose it. He refused. He wanted to be completely free, on his terms. He was not only fighting for his own freedom but for the freedom of millions of others. He fought for equality and would give his life for the cause. Few men embodied forgiveness, love, and grace like Mandela did.

I wonder if Mandela also continued to do things out of habit long after his release. How does one live as a free man after so many years as a slave? You see, when you are a slave, your master manipulates and corrupts your thought patterns so that long after you are free you still live as a prisoner. It is the continual, habitual pain that slavery pours on your soul. It is the body and soul that partners for an endless period. Eventually, acceptance kicks in.

WHY

Exodus 1:14 describes that the Egyptians "made their lives bitter with hard bondage." They did not really fight their bitter enslavement. Yes, they did cry out to God, but I do not think God responded because He felt pity. I want to believe it is because of His covenant to them that He responded. My guess is also that they were not able to fight back. Pharaoh may have used some smart strategies and strong military power. And the sons of Israel, originally being shepherds, would probably not be much skilled or have the experience to withstand any of these tactics. They come across as submissive, not even exploring the idea of being free. They did not even imagine the possibility. They were slaves and that was an unchangeable fact for the Israelites.

When I reflect on Mandela's life again, I did notice that he did not carry on with his life with a slave mentality. He came out of prison as a different man, full of remorse and forgiveness. But then I remind myself: he had twenty-seven years in the wilderness! The same wilderness that took the Israelites forty years to journey through. The same wilderness that I had to endure. The wilderness of leaving slavery.

I saw myself in the lives of the Israelites and of Mandela. I knew very well how it felt to be physically dependent and enslaved in my mind. I tried to run away from my harsh slave masters – the addictions I could not break, but my circumstances did not change. Loneliness would not let me escape and I kept running back to what enslaved me in the first place. A slave does not have the luxury of planning the future. A slave is only there to survive the present, hoping to survive another day. Addiction is nothing other than being enslaved by some master or another. That master will control your soul and your body. When you experience prolonged bondage, enslavement, or addiction, you lose your will to fight. You survive and become used to the life of a slave. You make peace with it. It becomes part of who you are.

Trauma often create addictions and causes this ultimate feeling of: *"This will last forever."* We so often see children being sexually abused going back to the same people that hurt them in the first place. A slave only knows that which is habitual in their lives, even if it kills them. The Israelites did not have a choice but at least they knew what they had to eat, how their day was going to look like and what the Egyptians expected from them. They got used to being highly taxed and abused. They were stuck but did not do much about it. They also experienced that feeling: *"This is going to be my life forever."*

My family home was rarely my safe place while growing up. Conflict increased day by day, and I could not really do anything about it. It is very difficult to escape addictions if your circumstances do not change. My circumstances just got worse.

Being a young teenager that had been exposed to pornography was not easy. Your body and everything about you are busy developing but mine had already experienced things that was meant for adults, not for children. You feel exposed, as if the whole world is looking at you. As if you are standing in front of millions, naked. My days were filled with fear, anxiety, and depression. I was a young girl with serious mental issues. Pornography works with another slave master: shame, and shame is the most ruthless slave master I have ever encountered. My mental health was shattered, but when you look at the research I can understand **why**. I was not the only one, like I thought. Today there are millions of children walking around with severe mental health issues because of pornography viewed from a very young age. Our youth of today are struggling more than ever with mental health, and trauma is almost every time the root cause.

> *The porn industry generates almost $13 billion each year in the United States. 9 out of 10 boys and 6 out of 10 girls have been exposed to pornography before the age of 18; the average age of first exposure is about 11 years old.*
> *28,258 users are watching pornography every second.*
> *$3,075.64 is spent on porn every second on the Internet.*[6]

The people around me treated me as a much older child because I had two older siblings and because I grew up "faster." I was more mature in physical experiences, but not emotionally. Many children act older than they are because of pornography and sexual abuse. Being exposed to porn was and still is abuse to me. Some might not categorize viewing porn as sexual abuse but it sure is if it is not a child's choice. It was my *right to choose* that was stolen from me and that created so much trauma in my life. This type of exposure accelerates you to the next stage of your life, without you giving permission. During this uncertain time, I found myself in a relationship with a guy three years older than me. I always hung around with my older sister and became friends with her friends, and I was soon part of a social group much older than me. I started to drink alcohol and went out to clubs and parties and was exposed to situations that I pray my 14-year-old will never see. My father did not always approve, but he was not always around. Because of the ongoing conflict with my mother, I guess he tried to avoid any other conflict, too. He escaped his own life, and unfortunately missed a lot of mine.

I exchanged my *Roxette* and *Kylie Monique* for *Nirvana* and *Def Leopard*. My life became darker and darker as my soul suffered. I had a few escape avenues during my teen years and those were sports and physical exercise. I was raised in a home where sports were very important, and you were most likely to participate in two to three types of sport in a school. Netball (a version of basketball) was one of them. I loved it from a very young age and used those times on the court to get rid of all my anger and frustration. In this way I had an outlet for my pain. It was in the year that I turned 15, that we got a new Netball coach. I was thrilled and hoped that she had some new techniques and skills to teach me and the team. I was aspiring to be part of the school's first Netball team as soon as possible.

A Wolf in Sheep's Clothing

My new coach was also our new science teacher. She replaced an older teacher that had retired. Everybody loved her and she sure got along well with everyone. She was funny, cool, and very relevant to teenagers. She treated children like her friends, and what teenager would not appreciate such a teacher? She quickly made friends with my mother, with all my friends, and was soon part of our family. My parents trusted her and would often leave us in her care. I slowly started to trust her, too. She was very interested in me, in my life and my family life. She cared more about me than I felt my parents did. You see when I was called weird, she complimented my weirdness. When my siblings made fun of me, she defended me. When I did something different, she appreciated my differentness. I noticed that and it made me feel valued, something that I never felt in my home. I trusted her with my family burdens and shared my fears, my insecurities, and the loss I experienced with my parents' marriage that had deteriorated. She always encouraged me and became a supportive role model to me. She listened and she cared. Something that I really needed at that time of my life. We had a good friend/teacher relationship for almost a year.

One evening she asked my mother if she could take me to a cricket match. I also loved cricket from a very young age. I grew up playing cricket with my brother and his friends. And a game out to the big stadium was a treat, especially on a weekday. Normally that would not be allowed in our house. But my dad not being around, and my mother lost in her own pain, it was probably not a big deal. While we were sitting and watching the game, cheering on our team, she touched my upper leg softly and said, "You have beautiful legs."

I was taken back and for a second thought that what I felt in my stomach was not real. I knew how butterflies in your stomach feels, and I knew how fear feels, and what I felt was no romantic feeling. I felt nauseous. It was just a normal compliment, I thought. Nothing else. I did not make anything of it. But I felt very uncomfortable. I did not know that teachers look at young girls' legs. Out of the blue she started to light a cigarette and asked if I wanted to try. I could not ever recall her smoking, and again I thought it is weird for an adult to ask a child if she wants a smoke, but I agreed and tried it.

My boundaries were totally violated, and I had no watchman to warn me. The next opportunity she used was in the science lab at the back of our classroom. She asked me to fetch something for her and as I turned around, she was right in front of me, in my face. She forced me up against the wall and grabbed my bum under my school dress, pulling herself close to my body. I was shocked, speechless, frightened, and aroused at the same time. I had no clue what in the world was going on. I had no boundaries and did not know what was appropriate and what was not due to the pornography that had broken down all my walls. I knew I was trapped. *I froze.* From there on the violations and sexual abuse just escalated. I fled to my inner world and started to dissociate myself from what was happening and from what I felt. It was the only way that my mind and body knew how to protect myself.

I remember going with her to her family farm, her sister attacking me from nowhere, obviously furious because her sister brought a child to their home. I remember lying in an unknown bed crying, pleading with her to take me home. She said she will make me feel better. I remember my helplessness. She was supposed to be my friend. Unfortunately, she did not understand her position as teacher and mis-used her authority. Her own dysfunction and brokenness caused her to fall in love with me and my circumstances made me an excellent prey.

She had done a pretty good job grooming me. At that time, I did not know what was going on. Only years later did I understand the whole process of grooming and the small steps she had taken to gain a hold on me. Sexual abusers are most likely to be someone you know very well. It is the inner circle, those that you trust the most that hurt you the most. Rarely it will be the 7-Eleven owner or the school's bus driver. It is family, friends, teachers, pastors, and coaches.

So, what does it feel like to be groomed, you might ask?

"Grooming is the predatory act of maneuvering another individual into a position that makes them more isolated, dependent, likely to trust, and more vulnerable to abusive behavior. The goal is to prepare

the other person for abuse (for example sexual or financial) later. The first step the groomer takes is to establish a friendship and trust. The scary thing is anyone can become a victim of grooming – especially people with soft-boundaries or whose defenses are down. Because there is no prototypical victim, anyone can be vulnerable to grooming.

Grooming can feel exhilarating, at first. The predator employs attentiveness, sensitivity, (false) empathy and plenty of positive reinforcement to seduce their victim. For their own part, victims can be so enthralled with, or overwhelmed by the attention they are receiving, they will often overlook or ignore red flags that might alert them that the person who is showering them with that attention is somehow "off." Little by little, the abuser breaks through a victim's natural defenses, gains trust, and manipulates or coerces the victim into doing his/her bidding. The victim often feels confusion, shame, guilt, remorse, and disgust at his or her own participation. Equally powerful, is the panic that comes with the threat of being exposed for engaging in these activities. There may also be an overwhelming fear of losing the emotional bond that has been established with an abuser. The victim becomes trapped, depressed, despondent, or anxious and fearful of being exposed."[7]

Realizing and understanding this whole process in the later years of my life was sickening to me. Most of what followed, I wanted to delete, erase or at best deny forever, up until the point where God led me to write about it. He wanted me to put these dreadful experiences, days, and years of suffering on paper. How could someone do that to a child? And **why** me?

That is still an unanswered question I have. I also was not aware that she was gay, I was too young to notice that. She continually told me that she loved me. It was very disturbing to see an adult fall in love with a child, to the point where they would want to pursue their feelings and abuse them in a sexual way. She kept on saying that I belonged to her as if she owned me. *I guess she did.* She was manipulative, aggressive, and warned me that I would not be able to finish school if someone found out.

She became very overprotective and obsessed with me. She always wanted to make sure that I stayed with her and with the "relationship." She was constantly checking up on me. She would pop into all my classes, flirting and secretly doing and saying things so that the other children would not see or hear anything. But I was left with the disgust.

Being my coach in almost all the sports that I participated in made it very hard to escape this nightmare. I was a nervous wreck and always ready to fight. I created and formed an image of being a strong child and I always made sure that I protected myself, but I could never get that right. I was always on edge with everything around me because of the fear I experienced daily, especially my biggest fear of all - that someone would find out what was going on.

I could not speak a word about any of this. I had no vocabulary for this. I did not know how to tell my boyfriend, my mother or anybody else. How do you tell your mother if she is encouraging the relationship? I did not know how to ask for help or even to begin to explain this whole nightmare. I left my boyfriend out of fear that he would find out what is really going on. I did not want to hurt anybody. As time went on, I gave up and made peace with the fact that I was a teacher's pet. A teacher that I once trusted. A female teacher.

A significant number of females who sexually abuse children fall into the "teacher/lover group." I became part of the statistics of sexually abused children. I always wondered **why** a woman, and **why** me? What did I do to deserve this? I blamed myself, always. Was I being punished for watching porn? I was forced to do things that I did not want to do. I became numb to most of it. Before this nightmare started, I took a secret oath with myself that I would never have sex before I was married. All of that was demolished in a moment. After almost two years, I remember her saying to me: "You must have known that you are gay." I did not reply to her manipulative comment, but I knew that I was not gay, and I had no plans to be a gay woman in my future.

My goal was to finish school and run away where she could not find me. It felt like I would never reach my goals and dreams to be free. I could not see myself living like this for another day. My fight was an hourly one. For the first time in my life, I wanted to die. I did not want to live anymore. What type of life will I have if this continues? How do one live with this continual pain? I swallowed a few sleeping tablets in the hope that I would die but it did not work. I obviously did not take enough.

I was very desperate.

During all of this, I continued school, sport, exams, and homework like a normal teenager. But I was far from normal. I could not concentrate, remember, or focus on anything. I was "brain dead," physically desensitized and mentally overwhelmed by all the emotional scars. Emotional scars are those that take the longest to heal. I was covering up all the traces so that I can go on with my life without anybody noticing my shame and deep wounds. My whole being changed and more than ever, I felt the utter isolation and identity loss caused by this pain.

My parents were not aware of my change and if they were, they never spoke to me about it. I was a teacher's lover, and nobody noticed. I painted the cover of this book you are holding when I was 16 years old in my art class, framed beautifully by my mother. I was hurting and crying for help, but nobody noticed. The other teachers, my friends, nobody? Who paints such a dark picture? *A very confused and broken girl.* **Why** did I carry that painting with me for more than 25 years? I carried the pain for just as long with me.

Carmen Watt

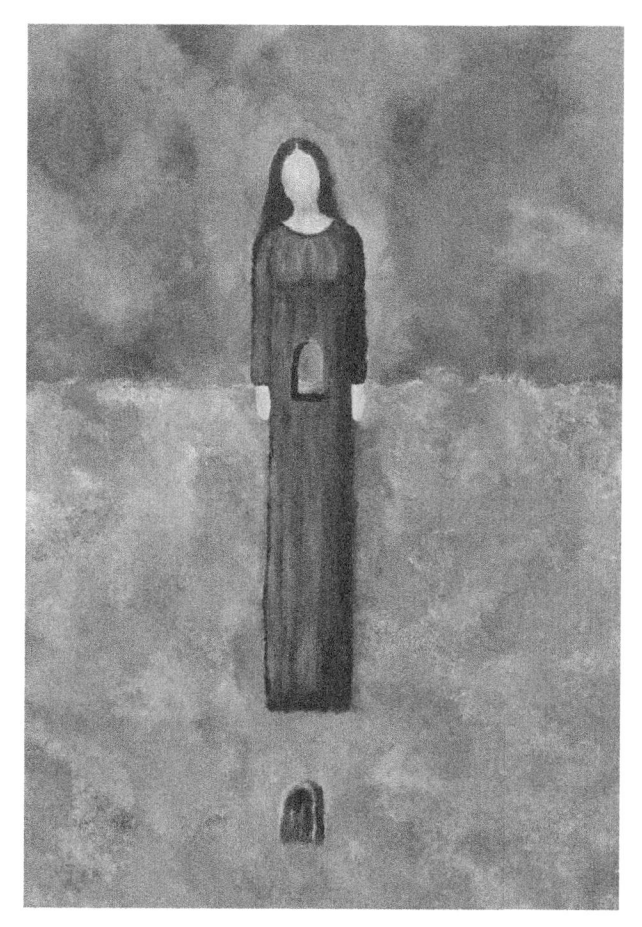

My note at the back of my painting.

Carmen de Wit 8 C
Dit dui op verkragting wat vir my
'n baie belangrike aspek in my lewe
is Ek voel baie sterk teen dit.

WHY

> *Translating from Afrikaans to English:*
> This painting depicts rape which is a very important aspect in my life and which I have very strong feelings against.

Maybe they did notice, but they just did not know what to do with it. It is easier to look away. When you looked closer, you would have seen a young girl desperately waiting, wanting to be saved. But there was no intervention at that time. There are too few people that act and stand with children that are being abused, too many people overlook **why** children act weird and rebellious, **why** they are "naughty" and **why** they act in dysfunctional ways. Parents do not see the "red lights" or warning signs of trauma. This dreadful and atrocious horror show lasted almost until I was seventeen. In those two years, I had seen everything and experienced everything. I will never forget the gay clubs she took me to where touching strangers was normal, and part of your "rights" just by being in the club. Being young and under-aged made me a prey for any such circumstances. I hated the fact that my body responded in a way that it seems that I enjoyed it. I hated the fact that I was not in control of my own body.

Again, my boundaries were demolished, and my body was not my own. I tried to escape, I tried to confront her, and I tried to defend myself, but I always lost. I was tired of fighting. I was fearful, stuck, and broken. I knew my voice does not stand a chance against her authority. I was emotionally dependent on her. I needed her. You must remember, when I had no one to talk to, she was there. When I felt alone, she was there. When I felt unloved, she was there, ready to listen, ready to care but slowly gaining ground in my soul. I loved her dearly as my "friend," but that all changed the day, she touched me. From there on until age 40, I tried not to hate her every, single, day.

I remember my mother found out just after my seventeenth birthday. *Took them awhile.* I remember the cussing and the anger that raged in my mother. Not towards the teacher but towards me. I was an utter failure and disappointment to my mother. An embarrassment. My father assured me that he would still love me, even If I chose to be gay. **Why** would I want to be gay?

No offense to any gay person reading this book. I just know it was not the life I was called to live. It was a lifestyle that was forced upon me. I wanted to have a family, a husband, and children. I grew up in a family. I value family, even though my family was broken. I did not see myself as being gay, ever. But my parents thought that being sexually abused by a female teacher while I am a teenager was different than when it happens to a child, and therefore assume that it was probably my own fault and my own decision. I did not choose it. Was it my fault? I believed so for twenty-five years. *But not anymore.*

My mother immediately went to the school principal. I was interrogated and asked a million questions that I could not answer. I was so fearful and afraid to say anything. I did not say a word. At this point, I already felt like it would be better for things to go back to what it was, because being exposed like that was far worse than the abuse, so I thought. That was only my slave mentality talking. Being abused was far better than the hurt I experienced from my mother. I was unacceptable to her.

Did you know that in a lot of cases it is impossible for a child to speak about the trauma and only with therapy can a child speak of the things hidden deep inside? Children create a barrier in their brain, unintentionally, to protect themselves. The language area of the brain can literally shut down, making it hard for them to share the words. That is the power of trauma.

Millions of thoughts flooded my mind all at once: *What will happen to her? Will she go to jail? Am I going to jail? What about my schoolwork? I do not want her to go to jail.* Irrational fear is the result of trauma.

It is this type of fear that gives us an explanation why between 90 to 95% of all sexual abuse goes unreported. Here is **why** I believe I could not speak, and **why** so many abused children will not speak either:

- It was too painful to talk out loud about such things.
- There is no vocabulary to explain such hurt.
- I felt ashamed and embarrassed.
- I was not sure how to talk about it or could not find a space to talk about it.

- I did not want my abuser to get in trouble.
- This was going to cause problems in my family/community/school.
- I am going to be blamed. (I experienced that firsthand.)
- I would not be believed.
- No one would take me seriously.
- I would hurt or embarrass myself, my family or someone else.

Therefore, it takes the average victim twenty-four years to reveal their secret and disclosure is often the key to recovery. *It took me twenty-five years.*

"Sexual abuse is the most underreported thing both in and outside the church — that exists," says Boz Tchividjian, a grandson of Billy Graham and a former Florida assistant state attorney.[8]

Even if it is reported, the abuser hardly ever gets what they deserve. They deserve the same amount of pain they caused the child, don't they? She only lost her job and was asked to leave. That was it. She got another job quickly after that at another school, repeating her same behavior without any consequences for her actions.

Just as I feared, everything came out into the light, and I was a humiliation to my family. I was not seen as the victim. It was as if my mother and the rest of my family members were the victims. As if I had hurt them or caused them pain. Sure, they were entitled to their own feelings, but what about me?

I blamed my parents for a very long time. I blamed my mother and who would not? I received no help, no treatment, no affection or understanding. Everyone carried on with their lives as they did before. There was not one conversation after that about anything that happened. I also had to go on with my life, but with no counseling or intervention. I had no tools to cope or no one to teach me how to process what I had gone through. As if my pornography burden was not enough, now I had to live with the scars of sexual abuse and my family that blamed me for being gay. How does anyone recover from that without any help?

Well, you do not.

You just live with it.

I just lived with it.

But the pain never went away.

CHAPTER 4

Fleeing from Egypt

"Your silence will not protect you."⁹

Audre Lorde

Living with that hurt was no fun and games. It was pure torture. But astonishing to see that when we look back, we recognize that we as humans are made to fight and persevere. Even when we are dying inside our inner being, there is still a possibility for life. Trauma alters the brain, but even now, I still think the brain is the most wonderful organ God ever made. Can I have my old 16-year-old brain back and rewire it without the trauma? In some ways, I think I can. I believe I can create new pathways for my thoughts that will help me to see my past and my future in a different way than I did before. Not all things can be as they were. I still struggle with the thoughts that I am a secondhand version of myself, used up in so many ways. But I also believe it can get better if you want it to.

Sexual abuse and trauma, much of which takes place out of public view, leaves deep scars that can cause a lifetime of emotional, mental, physical, and social dysfunction if left untreated. Research shows that chronic, complex trauma can even rewire a child's brain, leading to cognitive and developmental issues. Living with development issues is hard, but even worse is not to know who you are. It is so painful to wonder **why** you are here and what is the reason for your life. Nothing of what happened made sense to me. All that I felt was *"there must be something wrong with me"*. When you experience such pain, you will do anything not to feel it, to block it or even to develop certain coping strategies, and one of them I believe is, compartmentalization. We unintentionally put our hurt, shame, and pain in boxes. And we store those boxes very far away, hoping to never have to open them again. If it is for a short period, it is probably harmless but over time, it festers and it will end up erupting like a volcano. *Emotional silence is deadly to the body and the soul.*

Just before my final exam in Grade 11, my dad decided to leave his wife and his family. My mother hired investigators as she was desperate for the truth. She wanted to know why he never came home. It was a wild emotional roller coaster with my mother. But we found out why he never came back. Being exposed to the evidence and listening to recordings of my dad and his mistress was devastating to me. Again, when I look back, it was not the best choice to involve children in such a battle. I was still only a child, no matter my age. They were still my parents whom I loved dearly. My father left his family after twenty-five years.

As if I did not have enough to cope with, now I was fatherless. To see your father leave your mother for someone else is excruciating. He did not only leave my mother, but he also left me. It broke my heart in million pieces and the hurt poisoned my broken soul even more. I felt more rejected and poisoned with hurt than I have ever felt in my life. My family, my tribe, my people were shattered in million pieces. And we would never be together again. It is a pain and a loss that you cannot explain. I thought to myself: *Is he not going to miss me?* ***Why*** *would he leave me? Am I not important to him?*

All these questions are natural questions that children ask when one of their parents decide they want another life without them. Do not ever think you can have an easy way out of a marriage covenant. There will be damage. You can tell your children the most wonderful story about your separation, but when you break up a family, you chance breaking a child. They experience the damage, too. Children do not see their parents separately; they see their mother and father as a unit. To see that unit being divided and broken after many years was very hard. The sad thing about this situation was that I was still stuck with my life. My father had the opportunity to decide, and he chose another life. He chose to leave his tribe. He decided to create a new life for himself. With a new tribe. And I was not part of that tribe.

My academics suffered and I was barely making it. In my final year of high school, I decided to rectify my reputation, the little I had left. I decided to get myself the best-looking guy that was popular, the one all the girls would want to be with. I decided to fix what happened to me and to make sure that I was on the right path regarding my identity. I wanted to smother any rumors of me being gay and I went all the way to the other side of the pendulum to do that. And I found the perfect guy for the job. He was tall, blond, and very attractive. At this stage of my life, I knew exactly what to do to please people and I was determined to keep doing that. I was drawn to him although I knew it might not be the best route for me. I did not have a choice, I had to fix my life and I would do whatever it took.

At least my mother was happy her daughter was not gay after all. Anything **but** that. There were no standards in my life, no expectations, no planning for college, no dreams, no *"what you want to be when you are older?"* and absolutely no hopes for me as a person. *Nothing.* Only survival. I ended up in a very destructive and dysfunctional relationship. For three years, I was yoked to a very attractive guy who loved sex. Our relationship was built around that.

That and pornography.

That was the foundation of our relationship. Oh, and a lot of alcohol and drugs. There was little to no friendship in the relationship, and I slowly became used to being an object again. How did I end up in another nightmare? I fell into the trap of pleasing people, *again*. Pleasing people with my body was something that I knew how to do. That is the hard and very sad reality of some of the consequences of sexual abuse. It can go two ways: either you hate sex because of the abuse, or you have sexual addictions long after your abuse. You could also hate the gender who abused you. Or you could end up like me, very addicted to any sexual activity. Abused children tend to go back to what is familiar even if it is hurting them.

At that stage, he was all that I had. Our family had fallen apart, was dislocated, and destroyed. Everyone went their own way and continued their lives in their own box of pain. I believed that if I was going to survive, physically survive, I needed to stay with this guy. I had a false sense of safety in this relationship, but I did not know that. I lived in a world full of lust but lacking in intimacy. Intimacy makes you feel safe and valuable, but lust creates uncertainty and only feeds self-interest. It leaves you satisfied for a moment and very exposed the rest of the time. Lust is a thirst that cannot be quenched. Intimacy is secure, beautiful, and safe. It is a gift from God meant for two people in a covenant with one another. It is the one thing God intended for us to have with Him – ***intimacy.***

Intimacy is really what I was unknowingly searching for. During this relationship, my insecurities grew and my fear of not being wanted overwhelmed me. My hunger for safety only escalated. I would choose being abused above being replaced. Just do not throw me away. I was a master slave. Do with me what you want but just please do not leave me. *What a pity-full sight if I might say so myself.*

Rejection is evil to its core. Rejection is one of the most devastating emotional wounds one can experience, and rejection causes a traumatic ripple effect in one's life. It has the ability to blur your vision so that you are not able to see straight, especially when sexual activity is involved. All the lines were crossed and many times there were no lines. He cheated on me multiple times and every time I took him back, only too glad to, if it meant I was not alone. Alone meant being not good enough, not of use anymore and I feared that with my life.

I did not know my worth as a person. It was robbed from me. *I was identity-less.* The sexual abuse created a belief in me that I deserve to be treated like this. It is my fault. It is my fault if someone cheats on me. It is my fault if they abuse me. It was my fault if I was treated like an object. I never thought that it might be the other person's problem or wrong doings. I was wrapped up in guilt and fear. It was a humiliation to be the woman in my shoes.

I was so confused about life and where I fit in. My suffering became so intense that I finally decided to leave this blond hunk, for good. I had enough. I could not stand the abuse and neglect anymore. I knew I had to leave, or this life would kill me.

Never To Return

One of my passions is traveling. From a young age, my father exposed us to different countries and different cultures. It left a huge imprint on my heart. I decided to move abroad, work, and save money to make something out of my life. I had England in mind and applied for my working/holiday visa. Miraculously a friend sponsored my visa. At that time (1999), you had to show R20 000 South African rand (about $1,400.00 American dollars) in your bank account to receive a travel/working visa for two years. I will forever be grateful to my friend.

In January 2000, I left for good, and I intended to never come back. I ran away. I ran away from everything and everyone that had ever hurt me. I never wanted to see any of them again. I ran away from my own family as well. I remember my last farewell party and my last evening out with my sister before I would leave for good. I also remember the guy I met while being out with my sister. It was an unplanned connection that was made in a very short period of time. He was different, and he lured me in with his beautiful brown eyes and his interesting conversations. I saw him only twice after that and enjoyed his company, but I was on my way, and I was not staying for anybody. Not for another man that would probably use me, too.

I arrived in London very determined, but very fearful and scared. *Yeah, determination and fear can go together.*

WHY

Only three days after I arrived in England, I was invited to go to a club in the heart of London with my newly made friends. Being in debt to my sister's friend for lodging me, I agreed to go. What else would I do? I did not know anyone and going out was a means to meet new people. And on the other hand, I never said no, to anything.

Guilt and shame always cause you to feel in debt to others. As if they can see your sin. You feel judged although nobody said a word. Shame will kill you by your own doings.

When I look back at the remarkable story of the Israelites, I can just imagine how hard it must have been for them to follow Moses. Here they were, a tribe of thousands of people following one guy. They must have had some trust in him! But did they have any other options? They were not even sure where they were going. And they left the country that was all they had known for more than four hundred years. I can just feel their fear and uncertainty. They were heading into an unknown place, not even sure where they would get food or shelter. It takes courage to leave old things behind, to start all over again. To begin again. That is not easy and no matter what your circumstances are, if you are stepping into a new season or new territory, it will always cost you something.

Interesting thing to note in Exodus 13:17-18 is that God led them on a longer route. Read it for yourself: *"When Pharaoh let the people go, God did not lead them on the road through the Philistine country, though that was shorter. For God said, 'If they face war, they might change their minds and return to Egypt.' So, God led the people around by the desert road toward the Red Sea."*

When reading this I can just imagine God having something else up his sleeve. He knows His children so well. He knew that they would change their minds and want to go back to Egypt. Back to their old lives.

God did not lead me to instant freedom, he led me to the source of my freedom. The same with the Israelites. He wanted them to meet Him. To know Him. But remember they were slaves still on their way to freedom and breaking a slave mentality is not an easy task.

Back to my evening out with my new "friends." This club was no small-town corner pub that you might have in mind. Those old, fascinating, rich-in-culture clubs you do find in England as well, but this was something else. This was one of those scarce clubs and rare experiences where a Holy God met an unclean girl.

That is the beauty of Jesus.

The Jesus I never knew.

CHAPTER 5

Standing in Front of the Red Sea

> "Running away from your problems is a race you will never win."
>
> **Carmen Watt**

When you are an 80's girl like me, you would remember the clubbing and rave season of the world, if that was your thing. Maybe you are much younger than me, but I am sure your parents can tell you all about that time. Those were the days when you only went out at 10:00 pm after a few drinks and arrived home at 6:00 am, having danced the night away. My love for music evolved as I did. It went from Celtic to Hard Rock, from Bon Jovi to Trance music, and it always had a way to uplift me in any situation. From the outside, the club we went to looked like a huge, old warehouse. It did not look like much when we stood in the queues outside to be checked before you could go in. This underground or "warehouse" club was probably illegal or secretly run. It was quite an adventure to stand and observe all those people from all walks of life. As we entered the club my mouth fell open and my jaw dropped to the ground. I had to stop to take in what my eyes were witnessing. My body was covered with goosebumps, and my hair stood up straight all over my body, as if someone had brushed me with a feather from the bottom of my feet up to the top of my head.

There were hundreds of people, some dressed in black, some in white and then others in costumes. Very interesting costumes. Some had very little on. There were angel costumes with halos and wings, devil costumes and some clubbers were even dressed in Disney outfits. I did not think that I would meet Mickey in a rave club. There were men walking on stilts and for a moment I thought I was at the circus. But as soon I heard the music, I knew I was in one of the biggest rave clubs I have ever seen. It was the most amazing earth-pounding music. My feet beneath me were vibrating, every sense of my being awake, and I felt the music flooding my whole body with the rhythm of this club's heartbeat.

This three-story club looked like an old, overused and very dirty fireplace inside. It was only the lights that made this place attractive...and obviously, the music. There were different DJ's collaborating to create the sound where hundreds of people danced for hours on end. But not without the help of drugs. *You must really love dancing and be extremely fit to dance for 8+ hours without any drugs!*

I was already a very hyper-alert person, but this club had put my senses in complete overdrive. I was struggling to focus and was overwhelmed by the evilness I felt in this place. It was the very first time in my life that I experienced darkness in such a way that I could tangibly touch it. For a moment, I thought I was in hell. I was horrified. I tried to calm myself down with no success. My soul felt lost, and I felt the utter desolation of being alone. I felt beyond scared.

But since the beginning of time, I was in *"Someone's"* mind.

You see, I was raised in a Dutch Reformed Church. It is a South African, Afrikaans church. A very conservative and rigid church. I never liked going to church. I hated it. I never understood anything, and it was way too formal for me and extremely boring. I could never relate to anything that was talked about in church. I only heard rules. Lists of dos and don'ts. Knowing myself and my life, I believed I was not worthy to be a Christian or to even go to church. I felt condemned as soon as I walked through those doors. I never felt good enough and I did not think church was for people like me.

But I have many memories of Bible reading at night with my mother. Telling us stories about the great heroes of the bible. David who slew Goliath, Elijah that healed a boy and old Moses that led the biggest tribe of misplaced people out of Egypt. Now Moses is part of my story, and hopefully, you will see that he is also part of your story. I knew the stories of the Bible, but I never got to know the

God of the Bible. He was far away and distant, and with all that had happened to me, unreachable. I knew these dark and evil feelings I felt had to come from somewhere. I just did not know the source of these dark senses. From a young age, I was very sensitive to spiritual things and always searching. My soul was always longing for something.

I remember my dream catcher above my bed when I secretly followed the American Indian culture of the Cherokees. My room was filled with incense and soft Native American background music. I wanted to be in a tribe badly and they portrayed family like no other culture I knew. I was always searching through cultures and religions to find my meaning. Always searching for peace that I was so desperately in need of. Always searching for answers. *Who and what am I?*

I knew I was experiencing something supernatural in that club, I just could not put any words to it. I doubted myself and thought it must be all in my mind. I went through all the possible reasons for my experience. I hadn't used the ecstasy that I was given by my friend, so it could not be the drugs. I was very scared of drugs because of how my body reacted to it. I always experienced "supernatural things," or you might call it spiritual things, under the influence of drugs. Other times, I would just collapse from my blood pressure that dropped, because of the chemicals rushing through my bloodstream. For those that use drugs, there is always the possibility of the dark side of the spiritual realm which can become a very real, spiritual experience. Darkness and light have always been enemies and will never sit around the same table. They will be enemies until the end of time. Enemies they will be, but fortunately there is only one victor in this story.

After only a half an hour in the club, I realized I had lost my group. I was so disorientated and frightened, I really thought that this club was probably the end of me. Regret started to flood my heart and I wished I had never come to England. I wished I had just stayed in South Africa, in that broken relationship. At least I would have been safe. Here I was alone, terrified in a club in England, hearing and seeing things that I could never have imagined seeing.

Pursued from Behind

At this point, the Israelites were just as afraid as I was. You see, Pharaoh and his officials changed their minds and went after the Israelites, wanting back their slaves. Pharaoh realized that he would have no servants. I do not think it was even necessary to ask them what they wanted to do. They would have gone back out of fear. Seeing the armies approaching they became terrified. The fear and uncertainty were too great, and they had not yet built up their trust in God, their slave mentality was not yet changed.

When you have an enemy breathing down your neck all that you want to do is get away. Run away, but the Israelites had nowhere to run to, they had the armies approaching on the one side and the red sea on the other side. Just picture that for a moment. There they were on the edge of darkness ready to be overcome by their enemy on the edge of entering freedom, but they just could not see it yet. God had to remove their blindfolds bit by bit for them to *"see."* Their darkness was from living in Egypt for hundreds of years and they forgot who they were…and they also forgot who their God was. Let us give them some slack for being terrified, you would probably be, too.

I know I would. I know, at that moment, in that club, I was terrified, too.

But just like God worked a miracle on the Red Sea, in that club, God was doing a miracle in me, too.

CHAPTER 6

Crossing Over

> "He chose me in spite of who I am."
>
> **Carmen Watt**

The feelings of loneliness and fear in that club were something that I will never forget. When you have no boundaries as a person, you are not always fully aware of what you expose yourself to. You are naïve and stupid. I exposed myself to harmful and dangerous situations without even knowing it, plenty of times. For those affected by trauma, they experience grey lines in boundaries. They have no clear sense of black and white, of wrong and right. I lived life without the benefit of those warning signs.

At that excruciating moment in the club, I realized my life was in danger. I instantly felt I needed to hide, as if something was chasing me. It is very difficult to describe what I was afraid of. It felt like a presence was following me, ready to devour me. I found the nearest corner, hid myself in it and immediately curled up like a little child with my head between my knees and my arms wrapped around my body.

The dark atmosphere was gripping my heart and I struggled to breath. I started to sob uncontrollably and desperately wanted to get away from all the noises and voices. Up until that point I was used to seeing and experiencing all sorts of unthinkable things. But this was something else. It was as if I was part of another *world* for that short period of time.

Something in me broke at that moment and out of utter desperation I cried out: ***"Jesus! If you are real and if you are really a God, where are you?"***

I had an unexplainable, supernatural, miraculous encounter with God in the club that night. I know for some of you that would sound unreal and impossible. Maybe you even think that I am crazy. That is okay. Even I thought I was going crazy. But if you believe it is possible, you immediately put yourself in a position where it might become real and possible for you, too. The possibility for a God to speak to me never crossed my mind. But He did.

He responded: ***"I was there. I am, and I will always be there."***

As soon as I heard that voice my lungs were filled with HIS breath. My spirit was instantly renewed, it felt as if something came alive in me. It was as if my heart was being resuscitated. Extreme heat filled my whole body from the tip of my toes to the last hair on my head. I am sure if you looked at me from afar there might have been flames jumping from my skin.

I spoke back to this mighty Voice while tears were streaming from my eyes: *"Please change my life. I do not want to live like this anymore. If you change me, I will give you my whole life and I will follow you until I die."*

> "For whoever calls on the name of the LORD shall be saved."
>
> **Romans 10:13**

In that moment, Jesus saved me. I was twenty years old.

At the age of twenty, my whole life changed. For as many years, I had lived in utter darkness and in a single moment, I stepped into the light. I stepped into freedom. I walked out of that club into my new life, never to be the same again. On my way back to the house, that I shared with other South Africans, I realized my eyes were opened as if I had been color blind up until then. It was like I had received special glasses that night. My senses were awakened, and I felt other feelings for the first time ever. I felt peace, joy and I felt like I was alive for the first time. It was not a joy from an external experience, not like a happy feeling after a delicious bite of ice cream. This was pure joy from within. From my gut upwards, I experienced joy. I wanted to laugh and cry at the same time. I wondered how in the world I could ever share what happened with anyone so that they could understand it fully. It was just impossible.

My hope is that between these words you might experience the utter joy possible in being saved and forever changed by a God who is so interested in you, like he was interested in me. Jesus really saved my life. My soul was rescued from darkness, and I knew no matter what happened, nobody could ever take my experience away from me. I experienced the Living God for myself. I had a supernatural life-changing moment that forever changed my life.

As soon as I arrived back in my room, I realized I did not have a Bible. I never thought of having a Bible. I did not own one and did not read the Bible. From the age of fourteen, I stopped believing in God, completely. I could not believe that a loving God would allow me to be hurt the way I was. I had distanced myself from God and was determined to create my own life, to protect myself even from Him. God was not to be trusted. When I was sixteen, I had refused to be confirmed in our very religious church. I stopped going to church and I had been adamant about it. I did not want anything to do with God, His church, or His stupid religion full of rules and regulations. **Why** would you stand in front of a group of people and declare your beliefs and promise your commitment to something you did not even believe in. It was a joke to me. So many fake people committing to something they should believe in, but never really challenged to live any different. I knew I was different, and I was not prepared to submit to brainwashed rules implemented by screwed up adults. My actions were again a humiliation to my family. But I just did not care anymore. *Church and God were not for people like me.*

So, getting back to me searching for a Bible. I had to look in everyone's drawers and closets and finally found a small red Gideon's Bible in one of the drawers. What is the chance of that? Maybe you have seen some of those Bibles in hotel rooms or in hospital drawers. The Gideon's International is the outcome of two men who wished to combine commercial travelers with evangelism. What began in 1908 as an association of Christian businessmen placing Bibles in hotel rooms has evolved into an expanding mission to provide scriptures to all people in nearly every facet of life. Obedience from two men gave me the opportunity to read the Bible and find the truth in there at the time when I had no Bible. I have wondered how many others have been impacted by that Bible, just like me?

I began reading the Bible for the first time since I was a small girl without having to close it in confusion. I always struggled to read and to stay engaged in anything, but this time I could not put the Bible down. Even though the font was very small, I could not stop reading. It is quite something to realize that you have been redeemed and forgiven, and that you are no longer separated from God.

It was still very new to me. I struggled to understand and comprehend everything I read, but I did not want to stop. I was eager to read more. I pondered on every second word I read. I chewed on it and had to clarify for myself if what I was reading was true. That day, I could not believe what I read in that wonderful Book.

He loves me, just the way I am. *Really?*

He died for me, so that I could be free and have an intimate relationship with my Father. *Intimate? How does that work?*

He came to set the captives free… *including me.*

Be born again.

Be baptized.

Be filled with the Holy Spirit.

Wait? What?

What is the Holy Spirit? I had never heard of the Holy Spirit. I realized that this key truth had been hidden from me. The rigid church I grew up in never mentioned the Holy Spirit. Many times, things are hidden from you, but not from God. Sometimes you do not understand your **why** and *how* questions, but later in life, God reveals some of those answers, while others you might never know. **Why** I never heard about the Holy Spirit is one of those questions. But He knew how He wanted me to meet the Holy Spirit. It is wonderful to find the *Truth.*

It is the "aha moments" I love most about my walk with God.

A week later, I decided to move into another house with less marijuana and drugs. God sent me a friend from South Africa who helped me and cared for me in a time where I had no one. I began to explore the Word every day and filled my thoughts with the words I read on the pages. I started to ask questions because I knew I was not alone anymore. I knew He was listening. Little by little, God started revealing the truths of who I was.

My self-gratification and addictive nature never stopped. In fact, my shame and guilt only increased because I now knew I was not alone anymore. But I had small victories along the way. And I slowly got stronger.

I celebrated 1 week *"clean"* ...2 weeks...3 weeks...4 weeks...

But my body was so use to the endorphins that were released from masturbation and pornography that I could not endure the withdrawal symptoms.

"Drug addiction and sex addiction have similar effects on the brain – both primarily influence the brain's reward system through a neurotransmitter called dopamine. When a person satisfies a need or desire that is vital to survival or reproduction, dopamine is released, causing the person to experience pleasure or euphoria. This reinforces the expectation of reward and increases the desire to engage in the underlying behavior."[10]

The new Carmen and the old Carmen were bumping heads at every corner, and my newfound believe system did not match my addictive behavior. I was looking for things to sooth me or comfort me all throughout the day. From a cup of coffee to a cigarette. I would rather smoke than masturbate or watch porn but then again, I did not know that both behaviors were only symptoms of a broken soul. I did not know how to regulate myself. I did not know how to get rid of my fear and anxiety. Every new situation, challenge or uncertainty brought anxiety upon me. I had to look after myself for a very long time and it can become excruciating painful to do that day in and day out. I only had a few methods and that is all that I knew.

I was fighting this beast within me with everything I had. The war became very real to me. Now more than ever before. I would experience extreme irritability, cravings, restlessness, and anxiety. I could not stand to feel like that, and I did not know how to handle all these difficult sensations. I just could not stop my old habits. It was entrenched in me, and I struggled to escape my own destructive habits. It highlighted my need for urgent help every time.

"Withdrawal is a characteristic feature of chemical addictions and reports indicate that individuals struggling with sexual addictions frequently report experiencing withdrawal after a reduction in sexual activity."[11]

I slowly grew as a "new" person, but I still had a long way ahead of me to go - not knowing how the future looked. But I had hope, and I guess when you have hope, you have a whole lot going for you. *Right?*

One thing I knew since I met Christ is that I wanted to change. Everything in me wanted to be just like Him. I wanted to love like He loved me. I wanted to be as beautiful, kind, strong and powerful as He is. At times that goal seemed unreachable. It was my own goal and burden I had put on my own shoulders. I did not know how this new relationship was supposed to work. All I knew was that I wanted to vindicate myself from my past. I wanted to fix myself, to be perfect and pleasing for Him.

Moving Forward

When I look through the window of my own narrative to the Israelites' story, I can see that God offered Himself to the people. He also offered them transformed lives, just like he did to me. He made it clear to them all that He intended would happen *"if you obey Me fully and keep My covenant"* (Ex. 19:5). God offered to transform them through an intimate relationship with them.

> *"Intimacy and identity would be born and grow in a covenant relationship with Him."*[12]

This was the foundation of His covenant with them. A transformative experience that would change who they were. He was offering them an identity shift. God led them into the middle of the desert to offer them a life so different, it was as if they had never lived before. And to give them freedom to choose. I did not understand grace and His love for me yet, and I do not think the Israelites did, either. I did not understand the covenant that I now had with Him. But I knew I could choose. From now on *I* could choose. But that did not make the choosing easy. And no one helped me to choose. No matter how many times I failed, I always kept on choosing to follow Jesus. I think that was the result of my miraculous encounter with Him. I knew I could never deny Him. How could anybody after such an encounter? But I knew how to deny myself and hate myself for whatever mistakes I have made and continually made. Every day, I would get out my whip (my self-hate talk) and strike myself with it, and after that commit to try again. I was determined to change.

My year in London was not all gloomy weather, hard work and loneliness. Since the day I met God in the club, I pursued different things. Things that were very new to me but things I started to love. I met other Christians *(they were very weird, and some are still very weird to me)*. I received my first gospel CD from a friend and found a small group of people who also loved Jesus. I also celebrated my twenty-first birthday and entered the life of real adulthood. But I was already an "adult" very, very early in my life.

I knew that God had a purpose for my life, and I was eager to find out what that purpose was. But being a "new" Christian can be a very dangerous thing. You are very susceptible to false doctrines, believes, teachings, and false prophets. Especially someone like me. Remember I was a very sensitive soul, wanting to fit in, to belong was always one of my biggest priorities, if not my main goal in every situation and in every relationship. I heard the term "born again" for the first time and thought that that is probably what happened to me. I might have been born again, but I was still a very broken person, and I had no clue who I was. My identity was stolen, and I tried to be who I thought I should be to whoever I encountered. I was rarely myself. It took me twenty years to become who I was at that time. I did not know that it would take just as long to be whole and to bring Carmen back to her original state.

A Carmen who knew that she was loved and valued. A Carmen that knew who she was and love who she is. For some reason, I thought that once I submitted my life to God, my life was going to be better, "normal" with less pain and suffering. An instant soup kind of thing. A quick fix like we all expect from the fast-paced world we live in. Yes, I knew there was hope, and in a way my life was better, but it was still full of anxiety, anger, and addictions. I did not yet understand freedom or how to attain it completely. I knew from the Word that I was free, but my soul was still deeply troubled. I guess, like the Israelites, I was in the Wilderness, and did not even know it.

Just imagine for a moment thousands of people crossing the red sea that miraculously opened with the staff of Moses. You know the story by now. But before all that happened, they were surrounded by their slave masters with no way out. After God protected them for that night with the Egyptians breathing down their necks. God gave clear instructions to Moses. Moses then spoke to the people and tried to comfort them.

"Do not be afraid. Stand still and see the salvation of the Lord, which He will accomplish for you today. For the Egyptians whom you see today, you shall see again no more forever. The Lord will fight for you, and you shall hold your peace" (Ex. 14:13-14).

Remembering hiding in that club that night, fearing for my life makes it so easy for me to relate with the Israelites. The uncertainty that they must have felt. They saw the enemy and had nowhere to run. The Egyptians were so many and all of them were armed. The only thing they wanted at that point was to go back to Egypt and that none of this had happened.

But then the miraculous happened:

"Moses stretched out his hand over the sea, and all that night the Lord drove the sea back with a strong east wind and turned it into dry land. The waters were divided, and the Israelites went through the sea on dry ground, with a wall of water on their right and on their left" (Ex. 14:21-22).

Oh, how I wish I could be Michael J. Fox in *Back to the Future*, getting in the DeLorean to instantly be with Moses when he stretched out his hand over the sea! God divided the darkness and light in my soul that night. He parted the waters in my life. He made a perfect way and safe path for me to find Him. He rescued me from the hands of my enemy. From the outside, it looked like my life was over that night, but my life had only started then.

He literally pulled me out of the gutters of my own life. Of course, my enemy also had a plan for my life but at the perfect moment in time, I stepped from darkness into the light Jesus purchased for me with His life. And miraculously, just as the Israelites walked through the sea, to the other side...so, did I.

I walked over to the other side. I decided to follow Jesus forever. That night God really demonstrated His power and sovereignty to me. God did not only rescue the Israelites, but he rescued me, and he can also rescue you. No matter where you find yourself. Trust me, He will find you. That is, if you want to be found.

The Israelites were victors that day. They did not see the faces of their Egyptian enemies again. They trusted Moses and they started to fear the Lord, but unfortunately not for long. You see, they came to realize that the easy part had been to walk across that dry land towards the other side of the Red Sea. When Jesus saved my soul, it was in a matter of seconds that I crossed over from darkness to light.

But to stay in the light and to experience real change, it takes time and a lot of effort. It means walking and wandering through the desert.

It is the habitual trust and surrender that makes the freedom walk less painful. And where there is pain, you will find Jesus there with you.

Right beside you.

WHY

CHAPTER 7

Stepping into the Dessert

"The best way out is always through."[13]

Robert Frost

The phrase "walking on cloud nine" became a reality to me. I experienced heavenly feelings and I never wanted it to end. Once I understood what God had done for me in the weeks that followed, I sang songs of praise and joy for many days in London. He truly became my salvation. I was determined to stay in this happy place. It was a euphoric feeling. It was a feeling of overwhelming happiness, joy, and well-being. It was better than any drug, drink, or satisfaction I have ever felt. I bubbled over whenever I spoke to someone about Jesus. I felt this warmth inside of me that I never knew. It is very difficult to describe the change I felt. But it was worth sharing with others, even when they seem to think that I was weird.

> "The LORD is my strength and song, And He has become my salvation; He is my God, and I will praise Him; My father's God, and I will exalt Him."
>
> **Exodus 15:2**

But sadly, my joy did not last long. As Pharaoh came after the Israelites when they left Egypt, so did my boyfriend come after me. And a couple of demons from Hell followed him!

I guess the enemy knows how vulnerable a "baby Christian" is. I was vulnerable just like a newborn infant who drinks milk and still needs their mommy. I had no nurturing or leading as a new follower of Christ. All I knew was I wanted to serve God with all my heart. My enemy sure had some sleezy plans prepared for me. You know, discipleship and mentorship are one of the keys to lasting change, or so I have learned through the years. Walking alone always make you a very soft target. Walking with other believers to point you constantly towards freedom is fundamental in growing to maturity. That is if you can find mature Christians to surround yourself with. Mature woman and men that display authenticity, vulnerability, and acceptance. Freedom escapes many believers because of trauma and hurt. Yet I believe it is the walking together, the living together that helps one another to find true lasting freedom and maturity. Together, we heal better.

Most of my early years as a believer were focused on religion and what I needed to change to be a "good" Christian. Most of my effort was to stop doing something. I worked on my "not to do" list every day. But I kept on seeing what I was not and what I lacked in this new "club" I belonged to. When I looked in the mirror, I fell short every time. That was tiresome. Who would accept me as I am? I was a misfit. Now more than ever.

My boyfriend got hold of me in the UK and promised that he was going to change, that he also wanted to change and serve this God I had met.

I know, what you are thinking!
Carmen, how stupid can you be?

Well, I guess God already factored in my stupidity when He called me to follow Him. I believed my boyfriend and I went back to South Africa, to him. At that time, I really thought that he was serious and that I might have influenced him to serve and love Jesus, as well. How wonderful would that be? *(Saving the lost at all cost, right?)* I might have the opportunity to have my first soul saved for Christ. I desperately wanted to have that check mark next to my name. I heard that this is something you do when you love Jesus. You "win" people over so that they can join your club.

I was very wrong. Again, I did not know how this relationship should look or how it plays out in real life. I did not know that my efforts and my self-serving hard work were not something that Jesus expected from me. I went from darkness to light, and then again from light to a barren and a very desolate wilderness. And it cost me dearly.

> *"Wilderness is life beyond redemption, but short of consummation; but the former seems ineffective, and the latter only a mirage. The promise has been spoken, but who can live by words alone? The hope has been proclaimed, but the horizon keeps disappearing in the sandstorms. And so, trust in God often turns to recalcitrance and resentment. Faith erodes with the dunes. Commandments collapse into the disorder that shapes daily life. And judgment is invited in to share one's tattered tent."*[14]

I came back to the same destructive relationship. The pornography increased again, and I fell back into the same old patterns. I was addicted and full of unresolved issues, but I loved Jesus. How was that possible? I knew Egypt still had a firm grip on me. **Why** else would I go back to my old slave master? Let me explain for those who struggle to understand, just like I struggled to understand myself.

> *"Addiction is defined by the American Society of Addiction Medicine (ASAM) "as a primary, chronic disease of brain reward, motivation, memory and related circuitry. Dysfunction in these circuits leads to characteristic biological, psychological, social, and spiritual manifestations."*[15]

WHY

My addictions definitely kept on manifesting in my life, **why** wouldn't it? I received no help as a child with these addictions. I was constantly driven by the reward of the addiction. That was the only explanation that made sense to me. In "church language" you would say I was in bondage or in chains, cuffed to my addictions. But **why** was always a question I had. ***Why** for so long, Lord?* For those of you who have been exposed to drug abuse or maybe know a family member or friend that struggles with drug addiction, you would find similar patterns in their life. Some are harder to break than others, but it all comes down to the individual person, because not one of us are the same. We all have different shortcomings and broken parts due to our past. Unresolved trauma makes it very hard to escape addictions. Maybe you started moving forward towards the Promised Land and fell back into your old ways of living in Egypt. Maybe you are currently struggling to leave Egypt. You want to leave, but you do not know how. *I know just how you feel.*

The burden I carried of this dysfunctional lifestyle became too heavy and I felt that I had failed God, that I was a disappointment to God. I was disappointing myself, for goodness' sake. I knew darkness and light will always be enemies. I came face to face with the truth, so I knew my double life was going to kill me, at some point or another. I was not yet introduced to another key truth that is necessary for people to heal.

My soul needed healing. My soul needed restoration. I needed help. I was just a small girl that needed help.

Your body cannot do it on its own. God's spirit is within you, yes, but the rest of you needs to be aligned and restored, too. And on my own I did not know how to do that. So, I ended up going to church by myself. I told you I was determined to follow Jesus until I die. I tried to be the best person I could be, working myself out of the mud and slums every day. That is what sexual sin against your own body does to you. It breaks you down, piece by piece. I literally broke myself down every day and God's grace came to build me up again every time. I kept working hard to meet the goals of my new Christian life. I read my Bible, listened to worship music, prayed, fasted, read self-help books. *Well, I tried but struggled to concentrate and struggled to finish it.* I even helped and served in church. But at the same time, meeting the needs of a sex-driven relationship.

I know, crazy.

It was utter torment to my soul. I came to realize that my life was nothing new or different; there are lots of woman and men going through this tug of war in life. This constant battle in your mind. These two different worlds that are competing against each other. I am just willing to write about it but let me tell you: You are not alone. It is OK.

You will find that you are always in between who you are and who you want to be and then also most of the time you really do not know who you are anyway! I was like a yo-yo being played with. I was still captive, still a slave. I was saved from darkness. I was plugged into the light, but I realized that the glasses I wore kept me blind.

Fear, my desperate need to belong, and sex had a firm grip on me. So, no matter how many times I went to church, how many times I prayed, I could not get rid of the cravings and the insatiable thirst inside of me. I needed to be loved, I wanted to feel loved, and I connected any sexual activity with love. I always lost that battle. That constant battle in my mind. And I am sure it showed on the outside. I was filled with anxiety and fear. My hyper arousal increased every day and so did the abuse. Inappropriate scenes flashed before my eyes every single day. I could be busy preparing lunch or cleaning my flat and those scenes would rudely interrupt my thought process. Images and experiences I saw and lived in as a 14-year-old would not go away. I did not want to recall those images. It forced its way into my mind like only intrusive thoughts do. I did not know that it was a trauma response.

I was torn between what I knew all my life and my new love for Christ. I had loved Jesus since that night in the club. Serving God and being full of pain and hurt was anguish for me. Jesus was the most beautiful name I have ever heard. It was holy, sacred, and precious to me. He became part of me while I was unclean, full of fear and a whole bunch of hurt. I could never comprehend this utter selfless love Jesus had for me. This love is still a beautiful mystery to me. I fall to my knees every time I think of His pursuit to rescue me.

Depression started to walk with me wherever I went, and I felt its power every morning when I could not get myself out of bed. Depression is without question the most common reason people die by suicide. Yes, I was very depressed with reason.

"Depression has been found to be the most common long-term symptom among sexual abuse survivors. Survivors may have difficulty in externalizing the abuse, thus thinking negatively about themselves (Hartman et al., 1987). After years of negative self-thoughts, survivors have feelings of worthlessness and avoid others because they believe they have nothing to offer."[16]

The hopelessness I felt was real. I did not see a way that I could ever be free or loved. I tried this Christian thing, and I was not any freer than before. I believed that nobody would notice if I was not around anymore. And I could not live with that torment of addiction for another day. The voices of darkness, failure and disappointment became too strong. I hated myself. I hated my body and what it did to me. I wanted to kill my body which caused me so much pain in my life. My body did not protect me. Maybe if I were not attractive like my coach said I was, she would have left me alone and found herself another victim. Maybe If I were overweight and ugly, I would not have had this dysfunctional abusive relationship. My poor body got the blame for all my mistakes. But I was truly sick and tired of my body. I could not even make it as a Christian in this world.

After a few months of this roller coaster of religion and sex, I tried to commit suicide again by drinking a handful of sleeping tablets, hoping that this time I drank enough. I did not want to be on earth for another day. But despite my second suicide attempt, I survived all the tablets *again* and woke up after two days. I did not want to survive but I did. I was a zombie for two more days, and unfortunately realized that I was still alive. Still alive, but I was barely living.

Somehow, I got the courage *again* to leave my old life behind. God's grace and His love for me were not willing to settle for mediocrity. His love pursued me no matter how many times I failed. *Jesus had some real patience with me.* I went to stay with my brother. He opened his home for me to survive and recover.

I spend most of that year in my small room crying hysterically in my pillow. Hoping for no one to hear me. I called out to God daily, because it was all that I felt I could do. I felt utterly alone, rejected, messed up and full of physical withdrawal symptoms. It was a daily fight. But my heart would be filled with peace and reassurance as soon as I listened to worship music or spent some time waiting to hear more from Jesus. I started to read the Word to soothe me instead of my old behaviors of soothing myself. That is when my first revelation penetrated my soul:

"I am the true vine, and My Father is the vinedresser. Every branch in Me that does not bear fruit He takes away; and every branch that bears fruit He prunes, that it may bear more fruit. You are already clean because of the word which I have spoken to you. Abide in Me, and I in you. As the branch cannot bear fruit of itself, unless it abides in the vine, neither can you, unless you abide in Me. I am the vine; you are the branches. He who abides in Me, and I in him, bears much fruit; for without Me you can do nothing."

John 15:1-5

I burst from anger, screaming:

"I'm not clean! What do you mean I'm already clean?"
"Don't just get rid of the branch; get rid of this whole tree!"
"Throw me in the fire."

"Burn me!"

"I'm no use for you God! Please just let me die."

I was very, very angry. I had so many emotions that I did not know how to deal with even one of them. I never got tools or help to deal with difficult circumstances. Feeling lonely was something I could not manage or overcome. Feeling angry and not knowing what to do with that anger was just as draining and suffocating. My anger was stored up in my body and without asking it would explode out of me. How do we as people overcome *those* painful feelings? How do *you* overcome painful feelings?

Well, my screaming, pointing fingers and anger did not upset God. He did help me to make peace with His offer that when I abide in Him, He will abide in me. I did abide in Him, but sadly, I did not always *"feel"* better. And because of my addictive behavior and my need for feeling safe, my addiction did not subside. I could not think straight without it. I already had no stimulants, no medication, no sex, no boyfriend, no pornography. There was no escape. It felt like I was back to square one, back to the drawing board.

ME and JESUS.

I pushed through my own awkward self and kept on going to church, alone and desperate. In 2002, God led me to be baptized. I had read about it and knew that it was something I wanted to do. I just never felt "clean" enough. I know there are many people that think like I did. But no skewed perception or false beliefs could keep me away from freedom. I wanted to receive all God had for me. In Acts 1:8, it says, "You shall receive *power* when the Holy Spirit has come upon you; and you shall be witnesses to Me..."

I wanted that power. November 7, 2002 marked the day my old life was washed clean. *Finally.* I desperately wanted to be clean. I was on my way to true freedom; I could smell freedom. I knew my life would have meaning even if it had started off as a nightmare. My new journey of healing, grace and forgiveness began that day. I started to abide in Christ and He in me.

> "And I will pray the Father, and He will give you another Helper, that He may abide with you forever--the Spirit of truth, whom the world cannot receive, because it neither sees Him nor knows Him; but you know Him, for He dwells with you and will be in you."

John 14:16-17

Slowly but surely, I gained strength to face the world, to dream again and to fight for what I believed in. Jesus never stopped pursuing me. He captured my heart and soul. He was truly my first love. And at that time, He was my only friend. I must confess that music took the backseat. And everything that I loved dearly was replaced by Jesus. Again, I moved to the other side of the pendulum doing everything in my power to be fixed. I knew it would be not a quick fix, but I was still hopeful that my recovery would be quick and pain-free. I was not aware of the time in the wilderness that still awaited me. For some of us our time in the wilderness is days, for some months. And others, years. No matter where you are in your journey to freedom, never forget that you are not alone.

When Reality Knocks On Your Door

The Israelites left us with valuable truths that can change your life just like it changed mine. Remember after the Red Sea parted and the Israelites celebrated, they set out into the desert. Within days, the celebration ended as reality set in. They had no food. They had no water. An enemy nation attacked them, unprovoked. That does not sound like freedom to me. Yet they were "free."

Exodus 16:2-3 tells us: *"In the desert the whole community grumbled against Moses and Aaron. 3 The Israelites said to them, "If only we had died by the Lord's hand in Egypt! There we sat around pots of meat and ate all the food we wanted, but you have brought us out into this desert to starve this entire assembly to death."*

When I was a young believer, I always judged the Israelites. How could they be so pathetic? I mean really. Red Sea opening for them? Cloud hovering over them? They had God with them and here they were complaining about food and water? Really? They were so unthankful and such an unfaithful nation.

In my own life, even when I met God in the club and had that encounter, I would still fall back to what I felt was comfortable and safe. That was all that I knew and at that time, trusting God completely was not an option. I needed to be safe. I guess just like my addictions were controlling me, so did food and comforts control the Israelites. That is very short sighted, but slavery does that to you. You are only concerned with the next fix, the next meal, the next drink. Let's be honest, their basic needs were their only concern. Addictions are very similar. The only thing you can think of is pleasing that need that arises within you at that moment. Many people do not understand the root of that need.

The Israelites were happy just to survive and have their three meals a day. Their immediate gratification was like my own immediate gratification. It is absurd if you think that the God of the universe was caring for them supernaturally, and here you have a bunch of people complaining about their next meal. I do not judge them anymore, and I hope you don't, either. I guess I was hoping and trusting for a quick fix myself. At times, don't we all just want to get over hardship faster? Believe that if things would mend quicker than life can be easier, just a little bit easier? All they wanted was to speed things up and to get into the Promised Land. So yes, sad to say, even after witnessing God's awesome power against their earthly ruler, the Pharaoh of Egypt, the people were still not able to trust that they were destined for better lives.

They were stuck with their slave mentality. The result of this slave mentality was instability in their own lives. They were fickle. One moment they were uplifted by the excitement of the miracle at the Red Sea and the next minute, all has been forgotten; they might as well have been back in Egypt.

And as the Israelites and Moses continue to journey through the wilderness, there were more crises and challenges to overcome. In each of these challenges, the traumatic experience of life in Egypt influenced the response, which ultimately is the reason that a generation had to die out before reaching the Promised Land.

My own slave mentality made me unstable, as well. I never ceased trying to protect myself from any further pain. I made sure that my walls were high and my armor ready. My own armor I created for myself to protect myself, even from God. There were somethings in me that needed to die before I could experience true freedom. It just did not cross my mind that I would be wandering around in the *wilderness* just like the Israelites for many more years to truly see my value and to understand that I have a Creator that loves me unconditionally.

One morning, very early while writing this chapter, looking outside our window, where I was surrounded by beautiful grape vineyards as far as your eyes can see, I heard the Holy Spirit whisper:

"And for vineyards to grow some off the old branches need to die..."

Yes, a generation had to die.

CHAPTER 8

Trust, Denial and Failure in the Wilderness

> "Unless someone like you cares a whole awful lot, nothing is going to get better. It's not." [17]
>
> **Dr. Seuss**

During the years that followed, numerous times I was reminded that my name Carmen means: *"God's vineyard."* It made me feel valuable in a way and very aware of God's hand on my life. I had to make peace with the fact that God was working in *His* garden. Living around vineyards for the past three years has really impacted my life. The passage in John 15 that God spoke to me from years ago made complete sense once I walked through those vineyards and saw the branches that needed to be pruned. I saw the vinedresser taking the utmost care in every plant he planted, every row carefully nurtured and when the time was right, he had to cut back some of the branches so that it could create more growth and at the end produce better and sweeter fruit.

I saw that the vinedresser's soil preparation was one of the most important factors in grape farming. The soil of our souls also needs to be prepared, cleansed and at times, we need to break up the ground or "till it," as the farmers say. A vineyard cannot grow to its full potential without pruning. Cutting branches away in your life is not easy. It is painful, to say the least. It is more painful if you leave it. If you leave it, the only option that remains many times is to uproot the whole tree or gut it right down to the bottom. Growth and change are possible. That is if you want to see change. If you want to grow. If you want to get well, you can. If you want to be healed, healing is available for you. If you want to be free, freedom is possible. But freedom for the Israelites was still only partial because they were not utterly free. They still had to be pruned. So do we.

During my season of abiding and growing I was miraculously given a true friend, my life partner, my husband. That is part of my beautiful, but difficult life story. Remember before I moved to London, I met a guy? The guy with the brown eyes? His name is Wessel and I have been married to him for 18 years now. Let me quickly fill you in with valuable details of this love story. Because it is probably the best part of the story so far.

That night out with my sister turned out to be one of the most important days of my life. I saw Wessel from across the room. He came to introduce himself and we started a brief conversation. When I saw him, I was instantly crazy about him. There was something different about him. His eyes spoke to me. I loved our conversation and the connection we had. Unfortunately, I only saw him twice before I left for London. It was very hard to say goodbye to him. My mother told me secretly in our kitchen the day she met him that she believed I was going to marry him. I did not take what she said seriously, and my mind was focused on running away, moving on to a place away from everybody and anything that had hurt me. And I was not prepared to stay. Definitely not for someone I had only seen twice.

Being a new believer in London made me want to leave all that I knew behind and start over. I wanted a fresh start in life. A new beginning. Wessel was not part of that new start. I did not want anything to do with him once I met Jesus in that club. He phoned me, sent letters, delivered flowers from across the ocean. He kept that going for a few weeks. I knew he was serious about me. But I ignored him, and I ignored everything he sent me. I wanted nothing to do with any of my "previous life." I suddenly judged him and did not want anything to do with anybody unless they were a Christian. I thought only Christians were safe. I was fearful of my past. I never wanted to go back. *Yeah, right Carmen, and then you went back to your old boyfriend.* What a hypocrite I became in such a short period of time. That is what religion does to you.

I started to wear glasses with "bad" or "good" lenses. I started to label people. One thing that I hated, I unknowingly started to do too. I am sure you also know some Christians like that. I am sure I broke his heart. *I know I did.* I was too ashamed to tell him that I came back to a dysfunctional, abusive relationship, and not to him. In hindsight things would have looked very different if I had. But shame can keep us from relationships that are part of our healing journey.

As a young believer, I started to experience and hear God in different ways. I was drawn to the spirit realm and knew there was more for me to discover than what my eyes could see. After my baptism I had a very clear and surreal dream about Wessel crying to the Lord. He was lonely and full of despair. God showed me that I had hurt him. Not his ego, but the way I had treated him was detrimental to his soul and his trust in people. I wanted to ask for forgiveness. I did not want to be the reason for someone to *not* experience God for themselves. I tried to find his contact details. (This is before Facebook and the social media era.) I had to phone a few people before I got hold of his number. I was pretty sure after two years he was married already; he was almost 30 at that time. After a few days, I got the courage to contact him.

On January 7, 2003, two years later after our first meeting before I left for England, he was sitting in front of me at a coffee shop with his beautiful brown eyes staring at me, as if we were the only two people in the room. I was ready to explain my behavior and say my apologies when the Holy Spirit whispered to me: *"This is your husband."*

What?!

I thought that I must have heard wrong. How is that possible? *He is not a Christian*, I immediately thought with my judgmental and religious mindset. I was told not to marry a man with a different believe system as me. I did not want to repeat my history. Never, ever again. I knew what I heard, but I was very hesitant and scared. Fearful to make a mistake. We spoke for hours about the cross earrings and necklace I wore, why I love the cross and how I met Jesus. We spoke about faith, about the future and the past. Our friendship and love for one another was immediately rekindled. I was in awe and shocked to say the least. I was not prepared for what God had done in that one evening. God orchestrated a beautiful love story. The following Sunday in church, the Holy Spirit whispered in his ear that I was his wife. I know, what is the chance?

God loves to whisper. And I love it when He does. Trust me when you make time to listen you can hear more than what you think. Even now, it is my favorite story to hear him share with people. Every time he gets teary and remembers it as if it were yesterday. That whisper in his ear made it easy for him to stick with me in times when I drove him crazy. Six months later to the date, on June 7, 2003, we got married. In the heart of the bushveld (safari), surrounded by nature, the Big Five (Rhino, elephant, lion, buffalo, and cheetah) and big fires!

WHY

He is a very emotional and passionate person with a soft, kind heart that makes him a very understanding life partner. He never raises his voice and will never be abusive or cruel. That is a bonus for someone like me. At heart he is a very simple yet profound person. Give him a fishing rod, nature, God and his family and he is as happy as can be. He is selfless in nature and has a character of gold. Wessel is a very stable, strong, and secure individual, he always was. It was very hard not be intimidated by him. Who would not be? Up until today people ask me how I cope living with him because he is so perfect. That is what people think of him.

From the beginning I felt I was no match for him, due to my past, my addictions, and my trauma. I felt I could never live up to his standards. It was only much later in life that I came to realize that he wasn't perfect either, and that he too could hurt people. I was just always blind to his shortcomings. I only saw mine. I remember he told me before we got married that his father always warned him not to marry a girl who came from a divorced family. Wessel had his worked cut out for him in me. I was a lot more than a girl from a divorced family. I was a whole bunch of craziness. In my early relationship with Wessel, I subconsciously made him everything in my life. I found someone who will care for me, and I hung onto him for my very life. He became my safe place. Remember being safe was still my biggest priority. From day one, I was very attached to him and only later in our marriage would I come to understand that I had a very dysfunctional attachment to him. It is one of those patterns of attachment that are not very healthy and can lead to a lot of conflict. But thank goodness, we survived.

I wanted to be loved and cared for by someone. I wanted to feel safe, and I was safe with Wessel, deep down I knew that. It would take me a while though to realize it. I slowly started to believe that God really cared, and I felt God was saying to me the words he spoke to Jeremiah in the word:

> "Before I formed you in the womb, I knew you; Before you were born, I sanctified you; I ordained you a prophet to the nations."
>
> **Jeremiah 1:5**

He knew the end of my story from the beginning, and at times, I wished I could see some of it, too. This perfect love story was not always perfect. Our marriage was not easy. The first seven years were extremely difficult. I struggled to adapt to my new life, and *changes* were very difficult for me to process. We had normal differences like any other couple. Ours were just fueled by my anger, anxiety, and insecurities. Wessel had no recollection of these type of emotions and weird behavior. When I found him, he was a whole and healthy person. *So, I believed.*

In our early years we were not as educated in the effects of trauma as we are now. In those beginning years as a married woman, my life was filled with panic attacks, fainting, depression, and fear. My asthma inhaler was always with me. I developed asthma after the initial abuse and could not do sports without it. My nightmares continued, and Wessel did not always know how to help or how to fix the situation. I did not speak about it, either. I could not and I did not want to. And even If I could I did not know how to. Where do you start? Do you just blurt it out? Just thinking about it was too difficult already.

Cemented Thoughts

My sexual addictions and skewed thinking about sex also continued. I saw sex as the number one way of showing love and receiving love. That meant that my whole life revolved around that and all that came with it. That developed a lot of conflict between us, and it was very difficult to resolve it on our own. Complex trauma always has lasting symptoms and behavior, especially when left without treatment. Complex trauma is very different than a one-time incident. Complex trauma is multiple traumas that are very often extreme, ongoing and/or repeated. Some of these symptoms and behaviors I could not escape and others I forced myself and my body to cooperate with. I was very hard on myself, like I have always been. My heart remained turned towards God in my suffering and He, just like He did for the Israelites, made my bitter water sweet. The Word and my pursuit of healing were living water to me. God provided nourishment in every stage of my walk in the wilderness.

It was also the same for the Israelites as He built a relationship with them. He was continually providing for their needs. But not always as they thought He should.

They wanted to predict their outcome. They wanted God to do what they wanted Him to do. There is no trust in that. They wanted to control their circumstances to a point that it made them feel safe. Familiar things bring safety for people and yes, they were special people, but they were just humans like me and you. Feeling safe was a high priority for them. But God knew that. He was pursuing their hearts. Like he pursued mine. As He is pursuing yours right now, too. When we look at all the miracles that God had done for them, it is strange that they could not let go of their past and trust the God of all those miracles for their future. God never stopped being faithful. He cannot be anything but faithful. Trust me, I have seen in my own crazy life and marriage, Faithfull is who He is.

We decided early on in our relationship that we would always be willing to work on our relationship, and we would be willing to change what was broken or dysfunctional even if it took a lot of effort. But trauma, especially early childhood trauma is not that easily rectified. Still, I was willing to change anything that stood in the way of my healing.

Moses told the people: *"If you diligently heed the voice of the Lord your God and do what is right in His sight, give ear to His commandments and keep all His statutes, I will put none of the diseases on you which I have brought on the Egyptians. For I am the Lord who heals you"* (Ex. 15:26).

It was not easy for them to heed to the voice of the Lord. They could not get themselves to trust God fully, and their disobedience meant that some of them had to die in the wilderness before they could enter the Promised Land. Some things just cannot go with you into the Promised

Land. God is in no rush to get you to the Promised Land. He will do whatever it takes for you to get hold of the new life he has prepared for you. I knew God could heal, but every day I struggled with the diseases I carried from my life in Egypt.

Let us not forget, generations of Israel lived in Egypt. We are not talking about a few years. It was not easy for them to trust God, and many times they revealed remnants of their formerly enslaved lives. But then God always showed up and reminded them that He is their God. He was determined to have His holy nation, even today, He is still determined to find His lost sheep. It is always about His love for us.

And it was always God's love that bound Wessel and I together. His grace carried us in times when I had no answers to all my questions. And Wessel had more questions than both of us had together.

It reminds me of the words in Ecclesiastes 4:12: "One may be overpowered by another, two can withstand him. And a threefold cord is not quickly broken."

God was always the third braid in our cord (and still is today).

A cord that has many times convinced me that God is still pursuing me...

CHAPTER 9

Stuck with Egypt's Diseases and My Manna

> "When the alarm bell of the emotional brain keeps signaling that you are in danger, no amount of insight will silence it."[18]
>
> **Bessel Van Der Kolk**

I held on to this cord for dear life at times. Unknowingly, between this cord was thousands of threads of anxiety and fear woven into my soul. But I noticed I felt more and more comfortable with Wessel the longer we were together. Just being in proximity to him had made me more at ease. Many of my fears were being camouflaged by perfectionism, OCD, hyperactivity, severe allergies, depression, restlessness, agitation, constant fidgeting, and obsessiveness. I struggled to be around people, make appointments, introduce myself, build friendships, speak up and do normal things that normal people do. I preferred to be alone. That was easier for me to control. I thought I had a personality disorder. Definitely a mental disorder of some sort. **Why** am I so different? **Why** do I feel so different? Am I really that weird? What is wrong with me? These questions floated around in my mind every day. *I do not belong here* was a feeling that I could never shake off. I know now that many other PTSD survivors feel the same way.

"PTSD stands for Post-traumatic stress syndrome, for those who are seeing it for the first time. It is a mental health disorder that begins after a traumatic event. People with PTSD feel a heightened sense of danger. Their natural fight-or-flight response is altered, causing them to feel stressed or fearful, even when they are safe."[19]

That fear can last a lifetime. Many PTSD survivors live with a sense of "not being human," like an out of body feeling. In some way your body does not feel like *you*, as if your body belongs to someone else. It took every ounce of energy to focus on living and getting through a day, alive. I was not living. I was still only surviving. I was a mother at twenty-three with my first child. By twenty-seven, I was a mother of three girls already. I loved my children, and I loved every bit of being a mommy. Giving birth was one of the hardest things I had to do. Birth is a once-off event but raising children is a litany of small events every single day. I pushed myself through hard experiences combined with constant fear, every day. It takes consistency to be who they need you to be. I wanted to be perfect for them. It was at times difficult to be a mom to my kids who were then aged six, four and two. Three little girls with a mommy that had PTSD.

We had some fun in the house! Looking back, I realize that was not all that I was – a PTSD survivor. I am a very creative being and loved creating this perfect home for my children. I still do. The home that I wanted to have as a child I tried to provide for them. Having children was part of my healing journey. My disordered pattern of thinking said that I needed to give them what I did not have. *Safety.* I made safety, acceptance, and unconditional love my core goals for being a mother. But man, that song *Living on the Edge* by Aerosmith was my theme song. I was on the edge every single day. Striving to be the perfect mother, with my hyperarousal still tagging along.

Luckily, I had the opportunity to parent with Wessel. We made a strong bond and a steadfast parenting team, and he always blessed me by being a very present father with mutual values and beliefs. From changing nappies (diapers), cleaning up vomit or feeding the girls there was nothing that he could not do, and he was always willing to help me. He is the best father I have ever encountered.

All through my early marriage, I had to learn who I was. That was hard figuring out while you were a parent yourself. At times, I needed a parent. I needed a parent to tell me who I was and *how* to be a parent. To give me affirmation that I was doing good and instruct me when I needed guidance to do differently. I needed that. I missed that.

I knew from studying the Bible that we as human beings, made in the image of our Father (Gen. 1:26), are designed as a three-part being Spirit, Soul and Body. God made us three in one as He is three in one: Father, Son and Holy Spirit. And I knew I was filled with the Holy Spirit, but my body and my soul were still figuring things out. They needed to catch up. And fast. But they were in no hurry.

I slowly also realized that I was now a *Watt*. I belonged to Wessel. I not only have his surname, but I belong to him, and he belongs to me. I belong to our new family. I do not belong to my father or my family of origin anymore. *The Watts are my tribe.* Wessel and my children are my safe place, although I struggled to feel the truth of that for a very long time. I was always waiting to see when and who will leave me or hurt me next. I was always protecting myself, even from my own family. God's grace kept surrounding me in these "figuring out" times. He gives strength to those who are weak. He walks with the humble and He loves the true at heart. *Never forget that.*

Have you ever read in Exodus that the Israelites' clothing never wore out for forty years (Deut. 8:4)? I know that I wouldn't have enjoyed that, because I love diversity. But living in that miracle must have been amazing. But the question is, did they recognize the miracle when they were in it? Or is it just our human condition to continually miss God's miracles in our lives by instead looking to the future wishing for things to change, all the while missing the hand of God in the moment. Do not get me wrong, there is nothing wrong with hoping for things to change. But it is in the hoping and the waiting where we need to be fully present and experience God's grace in the moment. In my own journey as a mother, I saw that constant grace, never running out, that sustained me and strengthened me. One thing I found out about myself is that I love being a mother. I also loved being married. But being a wife to Wessel was another ball game all on its own. Life with a futuristic, creative, risk taker entrepreneur was not always easy. He is fearless and adventurous. We are such opposites, yet so similar. What I do not have, Wessel has and what Wessel does not have, I have. We always tried to look at life from a "team" perspective and always tried to avoid competing against one another, but he eventually became my mirror or measuring stick. I looked up to him.

We all know where comparison leads you. Still, he was all that I had. When I looked at him, I could only see my past, and how it ensured that I fell short in comparison. When I looked at him, I was confronted daily with my emotional inabilities, and any small situation would escalate into big problems and create a lot of conflict in our house. My behavior was warped and the smallest out of place object in the house would create a major blow up. When the smallest situation would go wrong, I would literally explode. My days and hours had to be planned and organized to the point. At this stage in my journey, I did not know the reasons for my behavior, I just followed what I knew made me feel safe, routine made me feel safe, like eating the same breakfast every day. *Silly, right?*

WHY

That is the beauty behind time in the wilderness, you learn a whole lot. Certain things, people, or situations I would avoid as much as I could, especially when I felt out of place, rejected and unvalued. I could not stand the feeling of rejection or the feeling of not being needed. I would lose my mind and any self-control I had when I experienced the smallest taste of rejection. Even if it was not the other party's intention. Rejection made me "see" things that were not always true. My lens was filled with lies. For Example, when Wessel made coffee without asking me if I wanted some, I would immediately crumble and experience feelings of neglect. I know it is dumb, but it is not dumb for the person that experience that visceral feeling of "I'm not important" and "He doesn't really care about me." It was instinctive. **Why** did I react like that? **Why** did I always feel left out?

It is a very real symptom of PTSD. Wessel might have known that something was wrong, but he was not aware of my trauma and the pain I lived with. He just tried in his own weird way to tolerate it. He would always encourage me to move forward. I remembered him saying: "*Focus on what is in front of you,*" or *"The past is in the past."* I knew there were things that were meant to be left in the past, but I could not get away from the past. I knew I wanted to avoid conflict but my behavior on its own caused so much conflict. I took baby steps, and at times I progressed but other times I fell, because there were just too many triggers that kept me in the past. You cannot move forward if you are stuck in the past. In my soul, I was still stuck in the trauma of ages 10-17 and could not bridge over to the other side. My life and my behavior made it very difficult to love myself. I somehow detached myself from myself, hating everything about myself. *Who would not?*

In our first couple of years together, I managed to escape the grip of pornography on my life. I was thankful and will credit it to my three pregnancies and all that it entailed. My focus never changed. Sex was still in the back of my head and deeply engraved in all my thoughts. It was the number one priority for myself and my marriage. I was still driven by the dopamine and the comfort it brought me. I could not really enjoy anything without it. I was to tense, anxious and hyper. I always looked very miserable to Wessel, and I guess it was somewhat true. I always needed something to make me feel better, to give that high and to take the edge off my life. Drug users experience the same torment. As do many people with other addiction too. Maybe you have experienced it as well. All of us at some point in our lives want to feel better, right? I needed to feel better and get rid of my pain *all the time.*

"The release of dopamine reinforces enjoyable sensations and behaviors by linking things that make you feel good with a desire to do them again. This link is an important factor in the development of addiction."[20]

I was constantly aware of my thoughts. At times feelings of desperation would grip me, and I just wanted to run away. I wanted to go to a place where I did not feel the extreme urges and impulses that comes with addiction. I wanted to hit my head against a brick wall. Yet, I knew what the Word said:

> "Flee sexual immorality. Every sin that a man does is outside the body, but he who commits sexual immorality sins against his own body. Or do you not know that your body is the temple of the Holy Spirit who is in you, whom you have from God, and you are not your own?"
>
> **1 Corinthians 6:18-19**

I felt like this verse was haunting me every single day. I stopped reading it. I could not apply it to my life. And I knew that I needed to apply the Word to my life. *But how?* When my addiction took over, my heartbeat would increase, a hot flush would fill my body, I had immediate tunnel vision and my brain would completely shut down. I was already over the cliff. And at that point nothing else mattered.

It was as if a snake constricted my mind with his sleazy body, slithering his filthy skin against my lobes. Suffocating my mind. And my body would not listen.

Many times, I cried out to God: "How can I sin against my body, if my body tells me this is what I need with such urgency?" The pain was so severe that I would only feel relieved, calm and at ease if I listened to my body. My body always won. I never managed to escape self-gratification or pornography. Some days I won the porn fight, but other days it beat me to it. It was always my medication to every ache or pain. That was the only way I knew how to medicate myself.

> *"Often when a child undergoes abuse or trauma there are not sufficient outlets for all the rage, despair and grief that results from the betrayal. It is simply too overwhelming. Sometimes there are also explicit or implied rules about keeping silent, leaving the child with no one to turn to for comfort. The child may place the needs of the abuser(s) or dysfunctional family members above his or her own needs, opting not to rock the boat. These emotions do not go away. Rather, they create an inner turmoil that demands self-medication, and without access to therapy or support, the wounded child may turn to addictive behaviors or substances to control the feelings. Self-gratification is one of the most accessible and available forms of numbing out, because you rely only on your own body to produce the intoxicating chemicals that soothe the pain."*[21]

I never could verbalize my emotions that controlled my behavior. I could not even say I felt scared. But I acted as a very scared person. And many times, I did not know why I felt scared. It was always a vicious cycle of my behavior and then the guilt that followed because I knew that it was not how I wanted to behave. My behavior got out of control, abusive and disrespectful towards Wessel. I had so much anger in me. It was hard to live with me. I knew that, acknowledged it, and would always ask for forgiveness. But I guess after a while it just became too much for him and a turnaround in our marriage took place at this time. I was thirty years old when my husband was exhausted and frankly fed-up with my aggressive and unstable nature. I did not blame him. He was ready to hit the road. He had enough.

He came up with an ultimatum: either I get help, or he would leave me. That is what was on the table for me. I was devastated. I could not lose Wessel or my family; they were all that I had. They were my life, my *tribe*. I did not want to be kicked out of my tribe. I knew how it felt to lose your tribe. I had pleaded with God for the most part of my life to change me. Some things just never clicked. I was never able to shift gears. On the surface things would slowly change but huge behavior problems were like fortresses built into my soul. I had some victories along the way, but I was always busy addressing the fruit and could never get to the root of the problem. It was very, very exhausting. All I wanted was to be fixed. I wanted to redo my engine. Pimp my ride kind of a fix. I wanted a new version of myself.

I decided to get help. Any help was a step forward for me. I started to read and do research on my behavior, and I took the step of seeing a psychiatrist. That year I was diagnosed with ADD (Attention Deficit Disorder) partially as the result of PTSD. I was told that my soul was like a chicken henhouse where I had laid all different kinds of rotten eggs. I was not diagnosed with depression or anxiety, all of those were only symptoms, but the main culprit was ADD. It was one of my *"aha moments"* in my life; everything made sense. I had a name for what was wrong with me. But my curious self immediately wanted to know what caused the ADD in my life or how did I get it? Was I born with it? Or did it develop in me when I was a child? I was determined to find out. I did not care how long it will take me.

> *"About 6 million children in the U.S. have been diagnosed with attention deficit hyperactivity disorder, or ADHD. Nearly two-thirds of those kids have another mental, emotional, or behavioral disorder as well. One of those conditions could be childhood traumatic stress. Childhood traumatic stress is the psychological reaction that children have to a traumatic event, whether it happens to them or they see it happen to someone else. These events can affect children's brains, emotions, and behavior in the same way traumatic events can affect adults. Sometimes, going through a traumatic event can cause real attention problems. But trauma, ADHD and ADD can be confused in diagnosis because the symptoms of trauma mimic those of ADHD and ADD."*[22]

God led me to a partial answer of what was wrong with me. He showed me little by little truths about my life. He took small steps with me just like a Good Father does. Patiently waiting for me to catch up.

God provided in small steps for the Israelites, too. He did not provide a month's worth of food. He did not show them what would happen in their lives in the next two weeks. There was no blueprint for their journey. God was the blueprint. He walked with them one day at a time. He was teaching them to trust Him.

Every action from God is a scene of His faithfulness being displayed. My own experience with God was just the same. We all want our complete healing or complete provision or complete breakthrough all at once, but God in his loving way knows that He needs to go slow with us.

Just between you and me, I think He knew the wilderness was best for me.

I was no different than the Israelites and neither are you. God is gentle with us but also just. He wants you to find your healing and to experience Him even in the baby steps. And yes, healing can come instantly for sure, or it can come in manna and quail every day, just enough for the day. When you are ready, He will provide more. But one thing I learned is, never assume God works the same with everybody. God is the same yesterday, today and forever, but we, His children are not all the same. Do not look at other people's miracles or healing, and then look in disgust to your own life. Only He has a unique blueprint for your life.

Coming back from that doctor for the first time, I felt over the moon and relieved. I knew there was something wrong with my brain and I immediately chose the medication option. God was busy showing me some reasons for my pain and He showed me that *I am not crazy*. There were reasons for my behavior. The hardest thing for someone like me, someone who loves to fix things and make things new, is when I cannot get something fixed. But that was about to change. I felt empowered and confident that I could change my relationship with Wessel and not be part of the statistics. Divorce was not an option for me. That medication changed my life in 40 minutes.

The medication, which is a stimulant that works by increasing dopamine levels in the brain. Like I mentioned before, *"Dopamine is a neurotransmitter associated with motivation, pleasure, attention, and movement. For many people with ADD, stimulant medications boost concentration and focus while reducing hyperactive and impulsive behaviors."*[23]

The medication changed my chemical levels and for the first time I really knew that I had been struggling with a chemical imbalance in my brain as the result of trauma. I was ecstatic and over the moon; it was one of the best days in my life. I was so grateful to God for rescuing me and giving me new hope. I was 'normal" at last. I could sleep. I could hear properly, no more multiple noises. I could concentrate. I was less impulsive and obsessive. The changes I have experienced were endless.

Wessel could not believe it. He had a "new" wife and we both had new hope for our future and marriage. Through his love and support, I learned to love myself and I was starting to except who I was and face the challenges I experienced as a person. I wanted to tell the whole world: *"See, I'm not crazy!"* At this point I never once thought of the sexual abuse or what happened to me. I never thought that it was behind my behavior. That was in the past like

Wessel said. All I knew was that I had a solution. And that was good enough at that point.

I still honor Wessel today, 18 years later for keeping at it. Never giving up on me. That is true unconditional love. The love of Jesus was displayed every day through the acceptance of my husband. It was not always easy to live with me, and surely it must have been difficult for someone who had no reference to sexual abuse and the effects there of. It was difficult to live with my own self.

I had a new view on mental illness. I would think twice before judging any person for taking medication for a mental illness. My old belief system, that was formed by my church, made me believe that medication was *"not from God."* I had always believed it was a weakness that made people sick and in need of medication. What a lie! Now more than ever mental illness is a reality for many people. I experienced firsthand that some illnesses do not disappear after one prayer. We will use prescription glasses to read better, but won't give our children medication if they need it? I believe every perfect gift comes from God and that medication was perfect for me!

Walking It Out

But when I think back to this time when I was between a rock and a hard place, I was reminded of Exodus 16 where God heard the grumbling of the Israelites. He never ignored them. He knew they were struggling. The poor Israelites kept complaining and wishing to go back to Egypt, back to slavery.

Becoming whole or finding healing takes effort. The easiest thing you could do is to go back. Go back to what you know. But it is in the uncertainty, the trusting and the holding on that brings healing. In the narrative of my story there were so many times where I just wished I could die. I told Wessel many times, I want to be with Jesus. I never thought that was a strange thought. Now I know it was my depression talking, *again*. The feeling of: *"I cannot live with this pain anymore."* I am sure the Israelites suffered from this kind of thinking, too. You must remember that leaving all that they knew behind was not an easy task and then they had to put all their trust into this one guy and the God who had sent him to save them. I felt compassion and empathy for the Israelites. Feeling unsafe is the worst feeling ever. They got on a path to the unknown. They were not sure of anything. Not even where their next meal would come from or how long this journey would be. At least I knew I had food, water, and clothing. But I know that some of you will agree that unconditional love, affection, and safety is just as life-giving as water and food.

The wilderness was an "in-between" place for me. It was a "not yet" place. What the wilderness does to your soul is a re-aligning with your Creator. A real fixer upper project, I would call it. Looking back, I can clearly see God was building my faith in Him, just like with the Israelites. He continued to provide for their needs, even when they doubted him. Even when they betrayed Him. Even when they kept on choosing Egypt in their hearts.

There are many people who will not experience freedom because of their unwillingness to trust God, and some will never see their freedom because they are unwilling to change. Some do not know how to change. Some never get the help they so desperately need. Some will not see freedom because they do not have a "Wessel" to walk with them to freedom, or they do not have a friend that will stick with them no matter what. The world today is evidence of that. Trusting God is not so easy for victims of sexual abuse. I know.

We struggle to trust people, even those that we love. It leaks into our relationship with God. That is why it is so important to find healing early so that your relationship with God and people can grow unhindered from the lens of the past relationships that have hurt you so badly. God intervened in this chapter of my life and I saw my medication as my manna. Only in a pill form. I not only saw that medicine as a life-giving miracle, but I saw God gently leading me in the right direction. Trusting God was not as difficult as it used to be.

But thank goodness, I did not have to eat that manna for forty years.

CHAPTER 10

The Law and Love

> "Great things are done by a series of small things brought together."[24]
>
> **Vincent Van Gogh**

My manna did not last very long, although I loved taking that small tablet every day. It was my sanity. And you better believe, everybody was better off when I took my medication. How wonderful to think the creation God made had such knowledge and innovation to develop medicine to save a life like mine, and many other people like me. Maybe you know of a family member or friend that you also believe needs to take medication. *Please do not tell them that!*

Medicine transform lives or ruins them. It can go both ways. It was as if someone pressed the pause button in my life, a moment in time where everything stood still in my mind. I had an opportunity to get my head around my life and my behavior. Finally, it was as if I was looking from the outside into my life. I was peeping through a window and saw much clearer what was going on. I was able to identify areas where work was needed, and my obstacles became smaller. I have to say that almost 70 percent of my behavior changed. Medicine fixed a lot of things, but it did not fix everything. It helped me to breath, to finally be able to think and focus. My flight and fight responses were more stable.

Sadly, I was still addicted. Medication did not remove that need or desire. Safety was still my priority. Sex made me feel safe. And Wessel's presence. For you, it might be food, your work or to be in control all the time. Maybe you need a drink every evening to help you feel calm. You might dive in your work to escape. Maybe you have a drug addiction. Every person is different. For some it is a "now and then" experience, for others it could be a regular dependency.

Intimacy was a high priority for me in any shape or form. I connected intimacy and love with an orgasm. That was my experience from a very young age. As a young child, I translated any sexual activity as intimacy because of my experience with pornography. It was part of who I am. It is quite liberating to share it with you. Maybe shocking, I know. But it is what it is, as Wessel always say. Some people connect their intimacy with a person, a thing, a hobby, nature, God, or their own dependency. It does not matter what it is. People struggle to name it for what it is. But not voicing it does not mean it is not real. Not speaking about it keeps millions of children and adult's captive. Voicing it can help people to be vulnerable and vulnerability is the first step towards healing. Voicing it will help you to find the root of that skewed behavior. Pornography and masturbation are controversial topics and are debatable to many. Even in Christian and other faith- based communities you will find very different opinions about these topics. But sadly, our children, your children will never be the same once they have been exposed to pornography, especially between the ages 9-16. Those ages are critical for developing children's identity. It is their forming years and viewing porn at these ages will have a long-lasting ripple effect. Effects that many adults and parents have no knowledge of.

I believe Church and faith - based communities do not have enough knowledge or insight into how to deal with sexual and pornography addictions, and the recovery from childhood sexual abuse. My hope is that this book will shine a light on the need for more people to come forward, more people that will raise their hand. And ultimately more people to help and protect our children.

Some people argue that masturbation is good for you. That it can be beneficial to your marriage. Nowadays pornography is just an add-on to have a thriving marriage. It is a tool to enhance your marriage, the media says. The world promotes self-gratification because there are apparent "health benefits." I believe everything can be debatable, but when it is the result of sexual abuse, your view changes and should change when you love and respect children. **Why** debate over something that can steal and rob your whole life? Go look at the lives of porn addicts. It destroys their lives and their families, too. It robs your whole life from you. It is just like any other drug. It eats away your soul. It leaves scars of guilt and shame that is difficult to mend. Over the long haul it will lead to death, the death of your soul. God created sex to be a beautiful expression of love from one committed spouse to the other, as a reflection of the intimacy that God wants to have with the church. Something that is very difficult to understand with our limited mindsets. It was not designed for you alone. I unknowingly craved intimacy from my Heavenly Father, a pure craving that was stolen from me through the sexual abuse I experienced. That core part of me was ripped out of my life. I never, ever spoke to God about it; I was too ashamed. I struggled to put sexual abuse and God in one sentence. As if He was not there. I felt embarrassed and awkward to talk to God about sex.

I did not have a correct picture of a father and therefore never thought of speaking to Him about that pain and hurt. I spoke about everything else *but* that. As if He did not know about my struggle to overcome this addiction that grew out of the abuse. I wanted to be closer to Him, but I did not allow it. How could I? And I did not know how to approach God.

So here I was torn between my soul and spirit. I was a double-minded Christian. I was free the one day, and a captive the next. One foot in Canaan and the other in Egypt. I was living in prison with a decorated cell. It looked beautiful, but inside there was a **war** happening every day. I attended Bible studies, listened to preachers, studied the Word, was part of small groups. I declared and proclaimed the Word backwards and forwards. Up and down. And sideways. I was still stuck. Better, but stuck. My body kept the score and I hated that it did.

Paul says in Romans 7:15-20, *"For what I am doing, I do not understand. For what I will to do, that I do not practice; but what I hate, that I do. If, then, I do what I will not to do, I agree with the law that it is good. But now, it is no longer I who do it, but sin that dwells in me. For I know that in me (that is, in my flesh) nothing good dwells; for to will is present with me, but how to perform what is good I do not find. For the good that I will to do, I do not do; but the evil I will not to do, that I practice. Now if I do what I will not to do, it is no longer I who do it, but sin that dwells in me."*

Sometimes it felt that someone else was in my body. It never felt like my own. I did not feel like my body belonged to me. The violation of my boundaries and my body made me feel that I belonged to everyone but me. That which I did not want to do, that I kept on doing. Maybe you have asked the question yourself. *How do you change? Behaviors? Mindsets? How do you get others to change?*

> "Don't copy the behavior and customs of this world, but let God transform you into a new person by changing the way you think. Then you will learn to know God's will for you, which is good and pleasing and perfect."
>
> **Romans 12:2 (NLT)**

My search for that answer drew me closer to the Word. In this season of drawing closer to God, He blessed me with a boy. One of God's many promises to me.

I was pregnant with my first child when I heard the Lord say: *"You will have a boy and you must call him Elijah."* I was like a small child waiting to unwrap this new gift. I waited quite a while.

After three girls, I thought that I heard wrong and maybe was a bit crazy. *Remember, I was a bit crazy at that time of my life.* I buried the vision and word from God but kept it safe in my journal. But my Father always keeps His promises. Even if it takes longer than what you might plan for, His timing is always as perfect as He is. Elijah changed my life and I never used my ADD medication again. He did not change my life because he was a boy, but something supernatural happened when he arrived that day. I felt closer to God and safer in my own body. My chemical levels were normal after the birth of Elijah. I nervously waited for the old Carmen and my old habits to resurface but it did not. I went back to my doctor and told him that I did not need the medication anymore. *I think I am cured.* He thought I was crazy.

But oh, the peace that flooded my heart when I held that boy in my arms. I could not wait for my midnight feeding sessions with him. It was as if God was with me in the room, every time. He brought so much joy into my life. That joy never left me or our family. His kiss on my cheek and his soft whisper in my ear: *"Mommy, have I told you lately how much I love you?"* Everyday. Every day he reminds me of God's love for me. Even when I have days that I do not love myself.

Never underestimate the power of children. They are powerful in the Kingdom of God and meant to be warriors with us as we do life together. That is **why** the enemy of God's Kingdom loves to hurt children. He knows the power that a whole child can carry. He knows when you hurt a child you damage their future.

In the following years, I constantly experienced God's favor, His grace, and His miracles in my life. Although we had persecution, financial loss and personal failure, just like any other couple or family does. God was visible during our suffering.

Let The Work Begin

I started to pour my heart and soul into ministry and community work – every church, every small group, every relationship. I gave everything I had to every person I met. Deep down, I wanted to love people the way I never felt loved. I wanted them to know that no matter where they are in life, someone would love them. Unconditionally. I wanted them to feel accepted, something I never felt. I was not able to receive any love back because I never felt that I deserved to be loved. Loving people was my goal. It was a gift that God gave me without knowing it at that time. The gift of suffering created in me a love for people that I never thought I had. I understood their pain. I felt it. I grew immensely in empathy because of my own hurt. But secretly, I wanted to give back to God what He gave to me, a second chance. I wanted to show Him how much I loved Him. I wanted to "repay" His goodness towards me. You must admit, I was indebted to God for giving me a new life. He was the only one who could love me. And still do. I owed Him everything. *That is what I believed.*

For many years.

I got stronger, better, and slowly started to believe that I was worth loving. I started to believe what the Bible says about God's love. I always believed the Word for others. I had immense faith for others and their needs but always struggled to believe the Word for myself. I never felt that it was applicable to my life.

> "See, I have inscribed you on the palms of My hands..."
>
> **Isaiah 49:16**

By age thirty-four, I started studying theology to increase my love and understanding for the Word of God and to equip myself for whatever God saw fit to use me for. Studying was never part of my scope for my life. I never thought that it will be possible. I was also a home-school mom that had my hands full with four children. I believed I was not academically strong and did not know if I would be able to finish one semester. The thought of being "stupid" was always part of my life. It was challenging to say the least. Studying was new and foreign to me. I felt incredibly inadequate at times and would redo things over and over just to make sure it was right, always doubting my own abilities. Wessel helped me through my essays, my assignments, and exams. Checking my spelling, my grammar, just like he did with this book. He was my cheerleader and still is. I could paint, a little bit, but write? That was very difficult. Especially being Afrikaans.

My second year went better, and I realized that I loved to learn and that it was something the enemy had stolen from me when I was traumatized during my younger years in school. I hated school because it was an environment full of torture and trauma, but I realized as an adult I loved learning, reading, and writing. I grew in different areas although it was very hard work. In the classroom, the new revelations of purpose that I was experiencing made me love God and His desires more than my own.

And yet, I still struggled to know who I was. I was willing to be whatever I needed to be to be pleasing to the Lord and the people around me. Even then, I did not yet realize that who I was, was not what I did. If you live only for what you do, you will end up as a very tired, burned out and used-up person because the busyness of life is a bottomless pit you will never be able to fill. If you live to perform and think that you should always keep up, at the end it will always shine a bright spotlight on your shortcomings and your weaknesses.

I was still wrapped up in a layer of anxiety and fear which I learned to manage through daily exercise (sometimes twice a day) by fixing others, helping others, giving to others, controlling my environment, controlling my diet, controlling my house, and controlling all situations as far as I could. When I tried to over-control, I ended up hurting the people I love. OCD was still very much a part of my life. But in a way, I thought I had become a "good Christian." I pictured those Christians that I saw when I was a young believer. They always looked so perfect, respected, and successful. I was working myself up the ladder, the ladder of holiness and approval, and I was proud of myself. Many days I thought, *"As soon as I finish my degree, people will value me and I too will be someone people will take serious, I will be "someone" finally and maybe I can also do something big for God, like what He did for me."*

"But we are all like an unclean thing, and all our righteousnesses are like filthy rags; We all fade as a leaf, and our iniquities, like the wind, have taken us away."

Isaiah 64:6

I never once thought that my deeds and my efforts were worthless. I was very hard on myself, only the best was good enough for me. I overcompensated in a lot of areas in my life and somewhere in the future, I knew that I would not be able to maintain this pace of performance. When I started studying, I fell in love with the Old Testament. But I never looked so carefully at Exodus as I did while writing this book. The Israelites were given the law on stone tablets and it started off with Exodus 20:2: *"I am the LORD your God, who brought you out of the land of Egypt, out of the house of bondage."*

Only after this first and most important words from God, do the requirements of the law follow.

God was reminding them who HE was.

Freedom was and still is God's first and foremost desire for us. Because of my filter of trauma and shame, even my Biblical studies made me feel worse about myself. I felt condemned. I was not condemned, but I sure felt condemned. I believed for too long that I was useless and a waste of space on this planet. I was always trying to earn my right to be here. Always trying to make myself "clean." And something that was supposed to free me, kept me in bondage. Whenever you read the Bible remember, God wants you to view and read the word through the lens of **freedom.**

The poor old Israelites kept going back to their slave mentality and behavior, even with the Ten Commandments in their hands. If you are a Christian and live with childhood abuse, the "law" by itself will not set you free. The Bible laying at your bed side table will not heal your wounds. The words on the paper are not what break the chains.

It is faith in those words that does. The Word has the power to transform your life, but first there needs to be renovation in your soul to be able to believe and receive it. Your actions and behavior will tell the truth, because they will be evidence of what you actually believe. It is the agreement of your soul and spirit with those words in the Word that has the power to flood your life with change.

Keeping score of what you do right and what you do wrong, what you have done and what you should be doing, is tiresome and will not bring you any closer to wholeness. Yes, it can help you to identify causes for concern, areas in need of growth, but to draw closer to God and fulfill your purpose as a child of God, you must restore your identity and your relationship with Him. You cannot restore your soul by your works. You can eat healthier and restore your health for sure, but restoring your soul needs a soul surgeon.

I remember the first time I read the Bible with a childlike mindset, knowing that I had experienced complete acceptance from Jesus in that moment and that Jesus would take me as I was. It was a profound revelation for me. I lost it along the way.

Looking back to my years in ministry, I saw that I had become trapped by trying to be a perfect Christian like those portrayed around me, and because of that, it prevented me from speaking to any people about my struggles and pain. *Especially not Christians.* This is only my experience, but I am sure there are more people like me out there. And there are wonderful churches, faith-based groups and communities that do leave room for people like me. If you are part of such a group of people, go and celebrate them. Take them out for coffee and thank them for being real and authentic. Thank them for valuing and accepting you. Truthful people and truthful conversations are rare.

Loving Jesus and living with addictions is hard, but does it have to be so hard to find freedom?

Maybe, just maybe, we are meant to find freedom...together.

CHAPTER 11

Golden Calves and Pornography

"Our lives begin to end the day we become silent about things that matter."[25]

Martin Luther King, Jr.

For a while life was good, as good as it could get. I belonged to a church community, I had close friends that loved me, and a wonderful family life. What more can you ask for? It was in this time of peace that I felt I had the courage to speak to Wessel about my addictions that did not just go away, like I thought they would. The longer I served God, the more I became holy and clean. Right?

It was only five years ago, at age thirty-five, that I had the courage to tell Wessel about the extreme burden I had been living with all my life. I prepared myself for two days in advance for this conversation, played the whole scene out in my head. I was a nervous wreck. I was so scared to be a disappointment to him or worst that he would leave me. It took me years to trust him fully and I knew it was time to let the monster out. I was hopeful, although very scared.

I shared with him in detail about my past, my addiction to pornography and that I still had a remnant of that left. He was supportive and valued my honesty. He listened and never judged me or blamed me. Unfortunately, he did not know how to help me, only to love me and support me. That alone was a big deal for someone like me. Acceptance is all that I craved. I realized I could trust him with my shame. I could trust him with my vulnerability. That was a gift. It was not that he was not trustworthy before, but I was not able to verbalize what was internally going on. I was not able to let go and trust him. Not with that part of my life. I was pretending to be in control, but inwardly, I was suffering. The root of porn and sexual addictions cannot be fixed by only looking to external methods to overcome it. It is a deep-rooted soul issue. The longer you stay silent, the harder it becomes to speak about it. Ironically, the more you speak about it, the easier it becomes. Remove the power from your silence and speak.

Addiction does not just go away once you tell someone. Those with addictions will know. On your own it is almost impossible, it can be done, but it is very difficult. That is **why** being accountable to someone is so important. That is **why** support groups are so valuable to society. That is **why** I believe family can help people heal. I used an app to help me see my progress and again I counted the days:

1 week... 2 weeks... 3 weeks... *I told you, I was not going to give up!*

Knowing my own struggles and past, I was very aware of the danger my children could face. We were very vigilant to protect our children, especially from pornography and any form of abuse. I was determined not to let any remnant of my forefathers, my past or any mistakes carry over to my children. I drew a line in the sand that day in the club. Every time I fell, I reminded myself that I drew a line in the sand. The devil loved to crawl over that line to make it seem as if there was no line.

Maybe you need to draw a line in the sand too. Do it multiple times, thousand times if you must; just do not give up.

I knew that my life could not be repeated in my children's lives. But I knew they were not immune. I was determined too always be vigorous and overprotective of them. We installed software for all their devices and laptops so that we could monitor and protect them from anything that was not appropriate and anything that has the potential to harm them. This specific software gives us a report and it blocks any site they try to enter that is over-aged. I recommend doing that if you have children. That is the least you can do for them.

But while I was busy, I was accidentally being exposed to pornography, again. I was testing a phone to make sure the software was up and running. I was proud of my achievement of being a few months *clean* up until that point. I did not type in the word porn, I only typed in naked. Naked is what I got. I thought at least it will take me to the meaning of the word *naked*, synonyms for naked or The Naked Chef, *Jamie Oliver*. But oh no, that accidental glimpse was a shock to my still fragile system. I could not believe how easy it was to view porn on a phone. How will I ever be able to protect my children? How does one fight against a culture of online pornography? It just seems impossible.

> *"Never before in the history of telecommunications media in the United States has so much indecent and obscene material been so easily accessible by so many minors in so many American homes with so few restrictions."*[26]

That incident was not just a quick, innocent glimpse. It was my biggest enemy greeting me with a warm welcome, *again*. I felt his nails cutting into my flesh, pulling me with force towards him. Again, I felt those warm and comforting feelings I felt years back as a child. I wished I had not seen those images. So many. I am still trying to forget images that flood my life daily. I immediately told Wessel about my utter shock. He did not understand the severity of the problem. He did not have knowledge about sexual addictions, and he sure did not know what to do to help me. He did not even know that he had to help me. Wisdom always comes after the lesson, but what happened that day was the same as giving a sip of alcohol to an alcoholic.

The lesson is, don't do it.

Wessel just brushed the conversation off with: "**Why** would anybody want to watch that filth?" My true thoughts were: "Seriously? The whole world is watching porn!" At that moment, I knew this fight was not over. It just started again, all over. I knew I was fighting a stronghold that was not prepared to let me go without a fight.

> For the weapons of our warfare are not carnal but mighty in God for pulling down strongholds, casting down arguments and every high thing that exalts itself against the knowledge of God, bringing every thought into captivity to the obedience of Christ."
>
> **2 Corinthians 10:4-5**

I pleaded with God to not let me go around this mountain again. In the previous chapter, we read about the commandments that God gave to Moses. Well, you might know the rest of the story. While he was on Mount Sinai with God writing out the commandments, Israel started to get impatient, and they asked Aaron to "make" them a god. That old Egyptian slave mentality popping back up. Unfortunately, Aaron was all too willing to comply. Exodus 32:4 tells us, *"And he received the gold from their hand, and he fashioned it with an engraving tool, and made a molded calf. Then they said, "This is your god, O Israel, that brought you out of the land of Egypt!"*

The children of Israel were still in the early part of their journey, and there were many lessons to be learned and obstacles to overcome. Most of these revolved around the fact that only God alone was worthy to be worshipped, and that they could not rely on themselves. What were they thinking worshipping a golden calf? Did they really replace God so quickly with a statue? Although God threatened to wipe out the people right then and there, Moses interceded for them. The children of Israel had already seen God do amazing things. But now they wanted him to do things their way and on their timetable. They were done waiting.

Their actions had consequences and their consequences led to death. A lot of them died that day! In fact, about three thousand died because of their behavior. But God kept on being gracious to them, and to me. He could have wiped them all out. He could have done the same to me, but he graciously kept on showing me my way to freedom.

> "And the LORD passed before him and proclaimed, 'The LORD, the LORD God, merciful and gracious, longsuffering, and abounding in goodness and truth.'"
>
> **Exodus 34:6**

When I was exposed to those images again, severe guilt flooded my mind. I felt dirty, unlovable, and cast out, all over again. I felt those same feelings I felt when the teacher touched me.

I was the scum of the earth.

Been There, Done That

I realized that I had pressed down the garbage inside of me instead of emptying the whole trashcan. This stronghold was still deeply rooted in my being. I just denied its existence. That is not how you fight your enemy. Denial and avoidance will keep you from victory. You do not run away from your enemy. You go after him, track him down, get a firm grip on him and kill him. Yes, I know the Bible says resist the devil and he will flee from you (James 4:7), but I am not talking about resisting combined with denial. I am talking about resisting combined with vulnerability. Look your enemy right in the eye and speak up about what you are struggling with in your life. Acknowledge what is torturing you. Name it for what it is and get help. Quickly. It does not help if addicts keep on thinking they are under a "spiritual attack." You are not under attack. Your soul is broken, and you have an addiction that needs attention. Whether it is an addiction, behavioral problems, or past trauma, get help!

In my own situation, I did not know of someone who would or could help me. How could I talk to Wessel again, if I am going to look like a complete failure? And I trusted him with only so much. I knew nobody with the same problems I had because nobody speaks out about these issues. What type of prayers did I need to be set free from this monster? I believe prayer works, but I did not think that prayer would work for this problem. Living with this opponent my whole life, I knew that saying one prayer was not enough. I had tried. And I did not want or need demons to be cast out from me, because that is the only thing Christians around me spoke about. I saw how they treated others like me. I heard their claims that addicts were demon-possessed or just needed "more of God" in their lives. Or the old, warn down directives: come to church more, pray more, read your Bible more.

Been there, done that, got the t-shirt.

I tried to speak to some of our close friends about sex, but the word "pornography" would not leave my mouth. I decided to keep quiet, ignore what is going on inside of my mind and keep on working to stay pure, holy, and pleasing to the Lord. The more I worked, the cleaner I felt. The busier I was, the less time I had to allow this lingering snake to suffocate me more. I was working to find all the people with the broken wings so that I can help them to fly again, while in my own life, I could hardly leave the ground. I was good at the ostrich move, putting my head in the sand. Hoping for no one to see me or my dysfunctionality.

We all have golden calves, don't we? Works was my golden calf. I made works and ministry my gods and bowed down to them every day. I wanted to work myself to freedom. The more I helped others, the better I would feel. The more good I do for others the more God will approve of me and hopefully set me free from my torment.

We have all made golden calves for ourselves at some time or other in our lives. Maybe it is your work, your sport. Maybe it is yourself. Maybe it is your body.

But that mindset of worshipping a calf in any shape or form has an expiration date.

CHAPTER 12

Wandering to Canaan

> "True happiness is not attained through self-gratification, but through fidelity to a worthy purpose."[27]
>
> **Helen Keller**

What is it about us as human beings that motivates us to build golden calves? I believe it is our skew mindsets competing with the truth of who we are. It is our brokenness that leads us to believe we need golden calves. Those golden calves can never compete with God's love. We can never replace God with anything. We were created to worship Him alone. On the one side, we have a people struggling to fully understand who they are and on the other side, we have this amazing grace that never gives up on us. Always persisting in His love, waiting patiently.

WHY

Yes, we know He is a jealous God. He did not want to share His people with any other gods, and He will not share you with any other god, either. No matter what god it is. But He will not force himself on you. He will gently show you who He really is.

I did not stop worshipping my calf and my torment continued. I wanted to ask Wessel to install the same software for my devices as well, but I did not. I could not confess my fear and shame to him. I was too scared of what he would think. But I was just as scared of what this addiction had done to my life and still was doing. I know what you might be thinking, *"Surely by now Carmen, you had to overcome this battle, right?"*

Nope, I only now realized that I needed stricter measurements to protect myself. I should have been treated like a child in this situation. I had to go back and rectify what I was exposed to when I was a child, by protecting myself now as an adult. But you know how the deceiver plays tricks on you, and he will do anything so that you stay stuck. How could I be thirty-seven and still have this *daily struggles*. At that time, I had finished my three-year degree, and surely, some or other time all that knowledge should set me free. Right?

Furthermore, I was receiving training to become a better counselor and mentor. That was my passion, to help others. I was a mature woman. I was a home-school mother counseling my children, teaching them Godly principles, Christlike character and demonstrating servant leadership. I lived in denial about my addictions all my life. As if it was not part of me. I never wanted it to be part of me.

I lived for helping others, but I could not even help myself. You see, it was the walls of protection around me that I had built around myself that made me carry this burden alone. Never isolate yourself from others, it is more harmful to your road to freedom than you think. There are many people that struggle with addictions, just not a lot of them will speak about it. Oh, how I wish for that to change. I dream of people standing up and speaking up against the pain and suffering that sexual abuse and pornography brings. Once I learned how to "read" other people's behavior, I could see their dysfunction, and I saw that I was not alone in this world of soul searching. There are many people stuck in their pasts.

If you know me, I am the person that will get up every day at 5 o'clock in the morning to go for a jog. I am the person that will eat vegetables straight for 21 days. I can read a book a day. I can fast for days on end. But when it came to sex, I had no discipline, self-control, no boundaries, and no protection. I compartmentalized sex. I had put it in a box where only I could see, hear, and feel the content. No one was allowed in that box. It was too painful.

- *68% of church-going men and over 50% of pastors view porn on a regular basis.*
- *Of young Christian adults 18-24 years old, 76% actively search for porn.*

- *59% of pastors said that married men seek their help for porn use.*
- *33% of women aged 25-and-under search for porn at least once per month.*
- *Only 13% of self-identified Christian women say they never watch porn – 87% of Christian women have watched porn.*[28]

I rest my case.

Here I am, so many years later in my life, living as a Christian, mother of four, still a slave to my own body. I cannot remember who I was at ten, eleven. I only remember images. When I look at Keenan, my eldest daughter, I know that I lost my youth. I am confronted yearly as they grow, with the reality of my life. The hurt at times is suffocating. I could not believe what happened to me. I was defeated by every realization of what really happened, and that devastation came in waves. Sometimes small waves, and other times tsunamis of hurt and resentment. When I got quiet and I had time to think, *which was rare,* I would sometimes close my eyes and imagine my daughters being 10...

Being 13, being 14, being 15...

I would put myself in their shoes, in their lives. Then the anger would rage up in me. How can anybody do that to a child? **Why** did I get hurt in such an awful, sexual way? That was one question that I asked a lot. **Why** was I stuck in my life because of someone else's wrongdoing?

God's Vineyard

I had all sorts of methods to deal with this pain that followed me everywhere I went. I started to drink more regularly so that I could not feel the pain. I exercised more to cope with the pain. My performance-driven lifestyle started to leave me unsatisfied. Most days, I would just try to forget and start over, begin from scratch every morning. I would run to Jesus whenever I recalled that He was with me and always my help in need. I would not speak about it, but I would cry about it. He knows my thoughts anyways, right? I wanted to be a good and godly woman. For my family. Most of my life as a mother was driven by the goals that I set for myself. I wanted to be the best mother, so that they would never, ever have to go through what I went through.

But deep down I knew the only good thing in me, was the Holy Spirit. His love kept flowing out of me regardless of my pain and my weaknesses. Experiencing the wilderness for such a long time has created a profound, deeper faith and trust in the goodness of God even when I wondered at times about my own brokenness, my feelings of being alone and abandoned.

Every new phase of my children's lives was a challenge for me. I had to be a mother for my tween and teen children without the reference of love and guidance from a parent at their age... I knew nothing. I had to overcome my own shortcomings, hurts and dysfunctions, so that I could empower them and develop strong women.

WHY

Here I was, teaching them about life, their bodies, self-worth, hormones, and sex. Surely God's grace was enough for me. *And his humor too.*

I have come to realize that not everything is awful or a complete lost in the wilderness. There is a lot of good that can happen while you are in the wilderness. Nothing in the wilderness is a waste. I learned to really love people and accept them for where they are at. It energizes me to help people in any shape or form. Helping and counseling others gave my life some purpose. And in a way kept me from focusing on my life and my own hurt.

God did eventually uproot me. You remember that I asked the Lord to pull out the tree and burn it? Well, I am glad he did not listen to me. But He physically moved our family to the Western Cape when I was thirty-seven. It is a whole different area in South Africa. For those who need to understand better, it is like moving from the West Coast to the East Coast in North America. It is two different worlds. De Doorns is a valley that is full of the most beautiful vineyards in the world. I knew I was entering Canaan. And it was right up my alley. Me being Carmen, being "God's vineyard."

I was just like the Israelites, those who were left at the end. I could not wait to have a "new" life free from constant fear and conflict, just me and my family, hoping my filthy enemy would also stay behind.

In the end, Joshua and Caleb were also standing on the brink of entering the land which God had promised to their forefathers. They were the remaining heroes, faithful to the end. It seemed my life was finally falling into place. I was thrilled that God finally decided to use this desperate vessel of His. All I knew was that I felt like I was being promoted, promoted to the opportunity for ministry, His ministry. *I was finally good enough.*

So, I became part of a ministry that served the community and helped to set children free. That is exactly what I wanted to do. Help children just like me. Help children that are being abused. But God had other plans for me. First, He wanted to set this child of His free.

Really free.

That is the true meaning of Canaan. Freedom.

CHAPTER 13

Running Out of Time

"Often it is the deepest pain which empowers us to grow into your highest self." [29]

Karen Salmansohn

I was delighted to move to a new part of South Africa and to be part of a team that served children. Wessel was ready for an adventure and was willing to travel for our businesses. We both knew, this was the right decision. We were going to take the leap of faith as we have done many times in our lives. This had to be our eleventh move or eleventh house that we had lived in during our then 16-years of marriage. This little town and its people captured my heart. Everything about their culture plucked on my heart strings. *And the vineyards, of course.*

I wanted to help in some way to fix our country's poverty, and most of all, assist the hurting children in these poor communities. The year 2018 looked promising, just like Canaan did, and I could not wait to be part of change. But if you want to be part of change, we all know that you yourself must also change. Moving cross-country was no fun and games, especially with four children and two dogs.

During my settling-in in our new town, finding my feet and adjusting to a new life with my family, I had more trauma training and got the chance to counsel more children. One of my desires was to train others about what I knew intimately, so that more people and parents could love and care for their children better. I wanted more adults to understand the effects of trauma on a child's life.

Even in wealthy first-world countries, there is a big need for healthy, mature parents to walk with their children. To lead them and to show them who they are. Children cannot figure out who they are on their own. We mold and form their identities as God leads us as parents. But a lot of parents do not know how to do that. They expect their children to figure life out on their own. We have children in the world walking around aimlessly, not knowing who they are or what they are supposed to do. They have no sense of belonging. Yet, they are part of families.

In this new adventure, I had to deal with my children's feelings of loss and uncertainty because of the move, and because their Daddy was traveling more than what they were used to. Him being away so often left me feeling alone, overwhelmed, and powerless. At times I would cry myself to sleep out of desperation and fear. The loneliness I felt was numbing to my system and I still could not understand **why** I felt abandoned and childlike anxious when he was not with me. I always felt safer with Wessel around and I always had this feeling that the enemy left me alone when Wessel was close by. *The beast was asleep while Wessel was nearby.*

In My Face

During this time, I was exposed to the extreme abuse of children and had to work closely with a boy that was molested by his father. After one session with him, his mother wanted to have a quick conversation about the situation she was in. I listened because that is what I was supposed to do. Counselors listen. What I heard in those ten minutes was a porn scene playing out in front of me. This mother was being used by her husband for other men's pleasure and he would film them. She cried and begged me for help, because she could not get out of this situation. How was I supposed to help them? I wanted to take them both to safety and care for them, but I had no power to do that, my family was waiting for me and it would not have been a safe decision for them.

I was only there to listen and for therapy for that beautiful, blond-haired boy. I ended the conversation as soon as I could and struggled to drive back home. I was shocked and nauseous. I felt exposed. Was this a sick joke,

I thought? I could not believe that this was what was happening just around the corner from my house. I thought it was only in porn movies that this stuff happened. I would know, I have seen it, but not in a small town in South Africa.

I was angry and horrified. I tried to share all the details with Wessel, but was overwhelmed and very emotional. I wanted to save that boy. I had to save him! I felt extreme pain, as if I was the one being molested and abused again. As if I was the one being part of a sick sexual relationship. **Why** did I feel their pain so intensely? It did not make sense to me.

And then, I received messages from this mother. Not one, but twenty or more photos of her, naked. She forwarded screen shots of messages between people where you could clearly see organized orgies. **Why** would anybody send this to me when I was there to help her and her son? Was it her cry for help or was it some sick joke the enemy was playing on me? I cried and screamed at the same time. I wanted to stab someone with a knife, preferably the father of that boy. At the same time, I felt shame and guilt, as if someone knew my past and wanted me to remember. My nightmares started again, and I could not get the boy out of my mind. I desperately wanted to help him, but the system did not let me. I did not see him again and nobody did anything with my information or the photos I had. I fell into a depression and my soul was aching for that boy. Who was going to help him? Who was going to save him?

I begged God to stop the people that hurt him. The "same" people that hurt me. I told God that it was going to ruin his life, just like it ruined my life. I did not get any response from God. I thought I would be a great counselor because I had experienced that pain and I understood it in a way other people who had never experienced that trauma could. I thought my empathy was a gift, and now it had turned against me. I had to learn that that is not the only requirement for a good counselor. That one incident brought me closer to my own pain and I knew I could not counsel another child that has been sexually abused, like I had – not when I struggled to come to terms with my own past.

It hurt too much.

You see when you experience trauma, "the emotions and physical sensations at that time are imprinted, not only as memories, but as reservoirs of disruptive physical reactions that can be triggered in the present."[30] It can be long after the abuse when unresolved trauma jumps out in a situation that has triggered that pain. I was experiencing my own abuse again.

Why *was I still hurting so much?*

It has been many years ago?

These were my questions I asked God when I laid in bed and I struggled to sleep. I could not connect the dots.

My forty years on this earth were coming closer, and I was not convinced that I would survive another forty years in this wilderness.

CHAPTER 14

Death in the Wilderness

> "Trauma creates change you don't choose.
> Healing is about creating change you do choose."[31]
>
> **Michelle Rosenthal**

It is the most painful thing to see and to experience, an adult sexually abusing a child. I would guess it is just as painful as losing a loved one or a friend that dies in a car accident. It just bruises different parts of our souls. Some scars are easily healed, and others linger for years. But I have come to learn that trauma is trauma, no matter what the circumstances.

I knew that the counseling experience with that boy was just the tipping point. From there on, it all went downhill. My life, and all that came with it, took a toll on me and my body. My body started to shut down. Literally shut down.

It seemed that my wilderness would never end. My body did not become sick overnight, but years of trauma and pain began to erupt like a volcano. I became physically sick. I was worn down, run down and tired. Very, very tired. I could not keep up with the pace I had set for my own life. Through all my wisdom, knowledge, and experience, I was still trying to fix myself in a way that I had to still realize was impossible.

I was stubborn in a way, I guess. I did not mean to be, it was just all that I knew how to do. I knew how to fight. And I did not want to give up. I did not want to disappoint God. I could not fail. I needed to be better. I needed to do better. I punished my whole being for letting me down. A lot of survivors of physical or sexual abuse hurt themselves by cutting themselves, starving themselves, or neglecting themselves. They want to escape the pain they feel within. I did that, too. I just beat up my soul every day. Nobody saw how I hurt myself, but I saw the consequences of that.

The truth is, you cannot love God and hate yourself. I could not protect myself, not from the abuse, not from the hurt and pain. And I unknowingly chastened myself for it. I did not love myself because I had failed myself. I had to blame someone.

Enough Is Enough

I finally went to see a doctor in the hope of getting some medicine to increase my energy. But instead, I was diagnosed with all sorts of ailments:

Adrenal fatigue, burnout, PTSD, stomach ulcers, hair loss, liver failure, depression, two autoimmune diseases, leaky gut, IBIS, viral infections, hypothyroidism, extreme allergies, anxiety…

The list goes on…

I knew my thyroid was a bit sluggish, but I was in total shock. I could not believe my body had betrayed me in such a way. I was angry and frustrated. Normal things I always could do became impossible to do. I wanted to exercise, I could not. I wanted to read, I could not. I wanted to see people, I could not. I wanted to serve people, I could not. I wanted to be my old self. *Whoever she might be.* In my desperate state, I would try to convince myself that it was all in my head. *"Mind over matter, Carmen, and focus."* Like Wessel taught me.

I wanted to get better as soon as possible but my body had just had enough. If my body could speak, it would have said:

Enough stress.
Enough trauma.
Enough abuse.

Enough conflict.
Enough shame.
Enough guilt.
Enough pain tablets.
Enough fighting.
Enough fear.
Enough worry.
Enough tension.
Enough "works."
Enough anxiety.
Enough escaping.
Enough revenge.
Enough sadness.

I went to the Lord in the hope of finding some answers, and the Holy Spirit whispered: "Now you rest!"

And I thought to myself: *"Rest, you must be joking, Lord. I do not rest. How do you expect a person like me to "rest"? That is just impossible! I am a goal-oriented person, a list maker, a type-A personality. I am on the go, highly driven and I like to get things done. I don't rest."*

Then I flooded God's ears with all my questions:

What type of goal is rest? And what type of rest, Lord?

Should I stop cooking?

Stop being a home-school mom?

Can I leave the washing?

Can I sleep until 11:00 am?

Can I stop being a wife?

Who is going to look after Wessel?

WHY

Can I quit?

Should I stop helping people?

Stop my training and my role in community work?

Answer me, God, please!

That same day, a wonderful friend of mine phoned me after we had not spoken for two months, just to share a dream she had about me. She was teary and emotional, and explained to me what she had seen in the dream. She said I was walking in a long corridor, and on both sides of the corridor, there were rooms. At the end of the corridor, there was this amazing sunny outside area full of swings and soft grass. My children were calling me to come and play, and I told them that I was on my way. But I just had to do one more thing. I disappeared into one of the rooms. The room was a torture chamber. She saw that I willingly laid myself down on a bed where I was then tortured, battered and scourged with whips. She did not see me fight. I willingly cooperated. I got off the bed, walked down the corridor and entered another room. I never got to play outside with my family. She ended the description of the dream by saying these words, words I will never forget:

"*I don't know what is going on in your life, but you are killing yourself. God wants you to rest.*"

I did not say a word and I asked no more questions. I rested. I was very sick. I had to drag my body out of bed and into bed. I had to sleep twice a day to survive the day and little to nothing could energize me. This was not depression. My physical body went on strike. She had had enough of this abuse as a vessel. Unresolved trauma has the ability to poison your body and if not treated, it is able to steal your very life.

People started to drain me. I could not bear to spend time with another broken soul. I felt crushed, defeated and extremely out of control. My children feared that I was dying. Overwhelming emotions of uncertainty hovered over our family. I felt weak. I was weak and I made peace with it. I canceled everything I normally did, and stopped everything I had been busy with, everything.

For the last two years, God had been pruning and cutting away that which was not bearing fruit. That is what happens in the wilderness. God refines you. It was extremely painful. But the pain did start to slowly subside. God wanted me to be with Him. He wanted to talk to me, laugh with me and cry with me. He is my Father and He wanted to heal my wounds, but He never got the chance. I was too busy "healing" myself...trying to fix my own wounds.

He wanted me to speak to Him about the sexual abuse and the effect it had on me. He wanted to hear me tell Him my story, because He cares. He is the best Counselor you will find. And he knew I needed to let it all out. All of the pain, trauma and abuse had to come out of hiding.

You see, He wants you and me to see the truth. The truth of who He really is. I just could not face sexual abuse and Jesus together. Maybe there are people that do speak easily about it. But it was always a conversation that I ran away from, even from the One who gave me another chance. Like the Israelites, I wanted to obey God most of the time, but I missed the heart of the Father every single time.

"They saw everything God had done for them – and utterly missed what it showed them about Him. They said "yes" to what they heard God saying – but utterly rejected what He actually said."[32] I heard what God was saying to me, but the trauma from my past confused me about what He was saying.

God wanted me to KNOW Him. When we know God fully, we can know ourselves fully. His heart's desire was for the Israelites, and for us, to know Him. God also wanted me to love myself as He loved me. I had to replace my self-hate with self-love, but I had never experienced it. I did not love myself, although others loved me. I had never learned to love myself. *How does one start to love themselves at my age?*

Nobody taught me to love myself.

I only knew how to sacrifice myself.

I had to experience the truth for myself. The truth of who I was. I was not yet aware of how to love myself. I had to rest to get to know my younger self and my older self, and to find peace in my past trauma.

Peace at last.

CHAPTER 15

Entering Canaan

"What we change inwardly will change our outer reality."[33]

Plutarch

At age thirty-nine, God was finished pealing the layers. He was gentle up until this point. He took His time. Like a surgeon opening a patient, slowly taking layer for layer out of the way to get to the main artery, he was gentle in reaching the places in my heart that caused me such tremendous pain. He was patient and kind. Year in and year out. He never rushed this wounded child of His. I never once heard condemnation from Him. Yes, from a lot of other people in my life, but never from God. I was only a child in God's eyes. And still are.

But think for a moment: How can a child love those who sexually abused her? How does one just forget and love their abusers? How do you love people that ruined your childhood and your body? How does a child get to that point? Who is helping children to love those evildoers?

Matthew 4 tells us that Jesus had to fight several horrific battles with the enemy Himself. He knows the wilderness. He was the first one who empathized with me when I had no one on my side. You see, I had read many books on forgiveness, sin, and healing. I had listened to hundreds of sermons on forgiveness. I have prayed many prayers of forgiveness. I forgave them. Multiple times. Every year. Every month. Every day. *I tried.*

I said it. I declared it. I even shouted it, but the pain and trauma would not leave me. I did not know how to let go. It was chiseled into me. I hated her. I hated my father, and I hated my mother. I wanted them to pay for what they did. They failed me and destroyed my childhood, something I could never get back. They did not protect me when they were supposed to. I never felt safe, and for most of my life I experienced extreme fear because of them. I wanted everyone that hurts children to be punished. They do not deserve grace. Hang them! Kill them. Even better, chop their hands off. The hands they were given to love, but instead used to damage and harm.

I had this inner *war* always raging in me. I told myself that I needed to love people because I was a Christian. I must love everybody. Because of the Word, I knew I was even to love my enemy. When somebody hurts you, you are supposed to forgive and if you do not, you carry unforgiveness in your heart. Then the wrath of God will be upon you. That is what I believed for many years.

That caused even more fear in my life. I believed that I did forgive them, but I did not know how to move on. My brain was altered, my personality was messed up, my body was sick, and my soul was stuck. I could not fix the mess; I have tried many times. I just wanted them to know how much damage they had caused me. How difficult my life was because of their actions? I just wanted them to understand and see. I wanted them to care.

Father, Forgive...

This past year, when our wonderful family took a 40-day tour of the United States, we attended a Christian Prophetic Conference. One special night during the conference, a woman of faith stepped into my life for a few minutes, and somehow moved the partition between my soul and spirit. She was able to shine a light on the main road to my pain. Not knowing her from a bar of soap, I was surprised when out of the blue, she asked me who had hurt me when I was fourteen. She saw right into my soul. It took me more than five minutes to utter the words; *my teacher.* It was the first time that my hurt met the teacher again. *After twenty-five years.* The woman said God wanted to speak to me about that.

I was sobbing and shaking and could barely speak. I have many times gone for prayer, hands were laid on me numerous times, but never had anybody shared such a word of knowledge with me.

> "For the word of God is living and powerful, and sharper than any two-edged sword, piercing even to the division of soul and spirit, and of joints and marrow, and is a discerner of the thoughts and intents of the heart."
>
> **Hebrews 4:12**

I was stuck, because I never spoke to anyone about it, and I could not release those who had hurt me in my past. I never had the opportunity. On my own I could not get it right.

God's grace and His power rushed through my whole being, and for a moment, I was with Jesus at His crucifixion. It was a spiritual experience I will never forget. By this time, I was already on the floor, kneeling in front of His cross. I could not look at Him. I saw my heart shattered in front of me for a moment, and then I saw what they did to Him. I could not believe the pain He endured. It was indescribable. I felt only the smallest bit of it, and I could not endure anymore of it. I could not bear to see Him suffer like that. The fire in his eyes penetrated my heart and I heard his soft voice whisper to me: ***"I don't want you to suffer. I have already suffered for you. I am the Judge. I love you. You are free."***

> "Jesus said, 'Father, forgive them, for they do not know what they are doing.'"
>
> **Luke 23:34 (NIV)**

I saw "her," my coach, in front of me, and for the first time, I had the opportunity to let her go. I never wanted to see her face ever again. When I saw her at first, I saw hate in her eyes. And I felt the hate rage up in me. I could not look at her. I looked away and Jesus asked me to look again. The second time I looked at her, I only saw pain, sorrow, and darkness. I did not feel hate anymore, I felt empathy, love, and compassion.

I softly spoke back: *"Father, forgive her for she knew not what she had done to me. Please do not hold it against her. She didn't know any better."*

Jesus could not bear to see me struggle in despair year after year. He grieved for his child who was stuck, while He had paid such a dear price for my freedom. I know He knew and still knows the end from the beginning. He saw beauty in all my hurt and pain. It must have been painful for Him interceding for me at the right hand of my Father for almost forty years. Pursuing me and my freedom.

But you see that is the beauty of the wilderness. The road with Christ has no time frame. A journey that could have taken the Israelites a few weeks took them forty years to complete. Some people are restored in a moment; others take years to unlearn what they have been taught, and finally to grow in wisdom and insight.

And perhaps the most important lesson to learn is that we heal better together. Churches, communities, and families should be your tribe as you wander your way out of the wilderness. That tribe that will drag you out of the wilderness into Canaan. The church is one place where

God can create an environment where people can be restored to their original image and identity...together.

Like I mentioned before, every child that has been abused experiences their pain differently. Every child heals different. Some become very strong and brave adults, while others stay stuck. But we need to at least give them a chance to heal. While I was on my road to true freedom, I knew God never left me, and I never blamed Him for what happened. He was not to blame. Many times, my places of despair were also the places where I knew God was.

Throughout my wandering in the wilderness, I never saw what I can see now, and I never knew what I know now. The truth of who I was could never penetrate my soul. It was really shame that had always separated me from God. As a believer, I was in Canaan with Egypt living in my soul, but I know now that it was not my fault. The abuse was not my fault.

I know that I am free, and Egypt has no place in my soul any longer.

Sin is not the cause of wandering in the wilderness. Love is.

And now, I had the chance to finally live in the Promised Land.

And so can you.

CHAPTER 16

The Grapes and The Giants

> "The ones who are crazy enough to think they can change the world, are the ones that do."[3 4]
>
> **Steve Jobs**

If you are reading this chapter, thank you for sticking with me through all these pages. I know it is a lot to take in. But I know my authentic story will help you to understand yourself and other people much better. I want to encourage you before we part with some fundamental knowledge. We all know that forgiveness brings healing, but it is crucial to deal with the pain and abuse in our soul and body. You might forget or want to forget, but your body remembers. Forgiveness does not always erase memories; it can, but it seldom happens. It is our responsibility to choose what happens with those memories. Your memories of the past can keep you prisoner to the past or they can become a point of reference, pointing you to freedom. You must bring your soul, body, and spirit into alignment, as God created us to live. We were created to fully hear, see, feel, and experience Him, through His lenses. Our real lenses. The lens of the Spirit. Living a spirit-filled life needs a whole soul. Otherwise, you walk around as a malformed, warped Christian. There are enough of those walking around. It is time for us to live real and authentic lives as believers. Community and the help of others makes it possible to heal from sexual abuse, or any trauma, for that matter. But I remind you that it is keeping silent that destroys you and brings death in your soul.

One of the key truths about Canaan is that you still need to work your fields, you will still need to fend for your life, and you will fight some giants, trust me. But it is in these times, that you must remember that you overcame the wilderness and that your time to take hold of your promise has come. Yes, the grapes are big and lush and available, but you still need to dress your vineyards. You still need to water your fields. You still need to cut off the branches that do not produce fruit. That is something that we all must do. Continually.

Freedom comes with a price. Jesus paid that price for our eternal freedom, but it is our choice as to whether or not we live in that freedom, now! Bravery and courage are needed to enter the Promised Land and to stay there.

Wessel installed software to protect me and our whole family. I am accountable towards him and myself.

Where we can, we try to be vigilant knowing that life is full of temptations and avenues that can destroy our children's lives.

Through therapy, prayer, healthy lifestyle, and the writing of this book, I finally felt safe in my own body. I had someone who walked with me through the process of what happens and can happen once you open that box of sexual abuse and start to deal with it. I had to learn how to stay actively engaged in my own healing and how to remain healed. Staying healed is something addicts struggle with and if you might be struggling in any way, do not feel dismayed. There is hope. When you find yourself close to Jesus, know that there is always hope.

My hyper-arousal is less and less every day and when I experience triggers or extreme fear, I can now recognize them better. I am now able to ask for help and I am also able to regulate myself in a healthy way. Fear of being hurt does not control me anymore. I wake up every day knowing that I have a tribe that loves me. I belong in this world. I belong in my family. But mostly, I belong to myself. I took the control over my body back from the hands of the enemy. I can love my body now.

Okay, I would love to lose a couple of pounds, but which woman would not?

I have the key to the door to my life and soul, and I choose who does or does not enter. I choose who speaks into my life or who does not. I choose who I listen to and who I do not. I choose who touches me or who does not. You can have that same key and the freedom to choose.

WHY

My illnesses are almost a thing of the past and that is a whole book on its own. But let me tell you many diseases can be reversed when you tend to your soul. Did my body suffer? Yes. That is **why** I now give it what it needs, and I listen to my body when it speaks. I nurture it as I should have. The soul and spirit working together in relation to your body is what encourages healing, restoration, strength, and inner grit.

When you belong to a tribe, a people that you can call your family, it is beneficial for you to live by the rules of the tribe. That creates a safe and secure environment for you. I still need to screen my phone. I choose with wisdom and discernment what I watch. I avoid movies full of violence, sex, and inappropriate behavior. If I have temptations and emotional challenges, I try to communicate it to Wessel. Our tribe does not watch porn. I listen to music that speaks life to my soul. And yes, I still love Queen and Bon Jovi. I still do not like watching cricket. Not because it hurts when I do, but because there are millions of other things I can do with my time. We all must be vigilant for the sake of our salvation. I choose to live in the light wherever I can. Even if I must stand alone.

Remember, at the end of the wilderness wandering, Joshua and Caleb were all that was left of the original tribe of Israelites who had left Egypt. No wonder they were encouraged multiple times, "Do not be afraid, be strong and courageous." They had to stand on their own to finish strong.

I turned forty while writing this book. It was a milestone for me. Not because of the age, but because I know that my time in the wilderness was finished.

Crossing Over

The year 2020 was a very difficult year for many people. Some people lost loved ones and others lost their jobs. Many of my close family and friends struggled financially and will probably find it very hard to get back on their feet. While many suffered, I was writing and walking my story out. The world stood still and so could I. Because it was time for me to write my story. To own my story. To do the very thing I had struggled with so much in my past. *It was time to say my truth out loud.*

It is time for you and I to invade Canaan and live in the fullness of what He has for us, without anything holding us back. Where are you in your wilderness? You might not be in a forty-year wilderness, but maybe you arrived in the wilderness in 2020. You might feel that your wilderness has been forever. I say to you what God said to Joshua when it was time to cross over, *"As I was with Moses, so I will be with you. I will not leave you nor forsake you" (Joshua 1:5).*

God will be with you. God will confirm his love for you over and over again. But it is not enough for us as believers to just follow God out of Egypt. We need to follow Him *into* the Promised Land. Is getting out of the wilderness easy? Not at all, it can be excruciating at times. But like I mentioned before, moving to Canaan takes effort, faith, and hard work. Dealing with your past and all of us have one, takes effort. Jesus is interested in our path to healing. He does not expect all of us to heal from trauma in the same way. That is **why** counseling and therapy is important.

Every counseling method does not work for everyone. People say journaling and writing is therapeutic, I believe it is, but it can be torture at first. To take what is in your head and then to put it in writing. Then to see it with your own eyes, makes it very real and very painful, especially when you buried it for so long like I did. *Do not do that!* Writing helps.

Talking about it in the beginning is not possible for some survivors. That is **why** I believe God led me to write this book. I found my own healing in these pages. I wanted to give up multiple times, but I stuck at it. I had Wessel that listened as I shared some of my memories for the first time. Memories that I did not want to have in the first place. I received proper support and care while I wrote this book.

Something magical happens when you write. It is as if the hurt and pain leaves your body and buries themselves into the pages. Trauma then has a way to separate itself from you. If you want to heal, start with taking a step. Get it out of your system. If it stays in your soul untouched, it will poison your body. You do not have to be a writer. Just start or find a friend and share your secret.

Restoring your soul is one of the gifts God has in store for you. No matter how long you have wondered in the wilderness. It is never too late. God will never treat you as a slave, though you might still live or behave like one. But that will only be the case until you become whole and fully YOU. The beauty of complete healing is it gives back to the abused child the right to choose. Our free will is the most precious gift to us.

For, always, the God who sets us free gives us a choice.

Choose freedom.

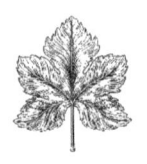

SUGGESTED READINGS AND RESOURCES

Trauma and Health

- Brown Brené. *Braving the Wilderness: The Quest for True Belonging and the Courage to Stand Alone.* Random House, 2019.
- Eger, Dr Edith. *The Choice Embrace the Possible.* Ebury Digital, 2018.
- *The Body Keeps the Score: Brain, Mind, and Body in the Healing of Trauma BY Bessel Van DER Kolk, MD | Key Takeaways, Analysis & Review.* IDreamBooks Inc, 2015.
- LEAF, CAROLINE. *Switch on Your Brain: The Key to Peak Happiness, Thinking, and Health.* BAKER Book House, 2018.
- Leaf, Caroline. *Think and Eat Yourself Smart: A Neuroscientific Approach to a Sharper Mind and Healthier Life.* Baker Books, an Imprint of Baker Publishing Group, 2017.

- Levine, Peter A. *Healing Trauma: A Pioneering Program for Restoring the Wisdom of Your Body*. ReadHowYouWant, 2012.
- Parks, Penny. *Rescuing the 'Inner Child': Therapy for Adults Sexually Abused as Children*. Condor, 1998.
- Perry, Bruce D and Oprah Winfrey. *What Happened to You?: Conversations on Trauma, Resilience, and Healing*. Bluebird, 2021.
- Perry, Bruce Duncan, and Maia Szalavitz. *The Boy Who Was Raised as a Dog: And Other Stories from a Child Psychiatrist's Notebook*. Basic Books, 2008.
- Toon, Kay, and Carolyn Ainscough. *Breaking Free: Help for Survivors of Child Sexual Abuse*. Sheldon Press, 2018.

Soul "Tools"

- Littauer, Florence. *Personality plus for Couples: Understanding Yourself and the One You Love/ by FLORENCE LITTAUER*.
- Leman, Kevin. *The Birth Order Book: Why You Are the Way You Are*. Revell, 2015.
- Chapman, Gary D. *The Heart of the FIVE Love Languages*. Northfield Pub, 2008.
- Cloud, Henry, and John Sims Townsend. *Boundaries*. Zondervan, 2004.

ADHD

- Berg, Hykie. *My Stryd Met Adhd: Die Onsigbare Oorlog*. Lux Verbi, 'n Druknaam Van NB-Uigewers, 2020.
- Kelly, Kate, and Peggy Ramundo. *You Mean I'm Not Lazy, Stupid or Crazy?!: A Self-Help Book for Adults with Attention Deficit Disorder*. Simon & Schuster, 2006.

Addiction and Pornography

- Foubert, John. *How Pornography Harms: What Today's Teens, Young Adults, Parents, and Pastors Need to Know*. LifeRich Publishing, 2016.

- Park, J. S., and Rob Connelly. *Cutting It off: Breaking Porn Addiction and How to Quit for Good*. The Way Everlasting Ministry., 2014.

- Fradd, Matt. *Delivered: True Stories of Men and Women Who Turned from Porn to Purity*. Catholic Answers Press, 2013.

- Wilson, Gary. *Your Brain on Porn: Internet Pornography and the Emerging Science of Addiction*. Commonwealth Publishing, 2017.

- https://www.covenanteyes.com/
- https://axis.org
- https://metoomvmt.org/

BIOGRAPHY

Carmen Watt is a speaker, writer, and author of the book, *Why; Sexual Abuse & Pornography: Daily Battles That Can Cause a Lifetime of War.* Carmen completed her ministry degree at Rhema Bible College in South Africa, and further educated herself in trauma counseling and how to walk with wounded children. After more than twenty-five years of PTSD, addiction, and pain as the result of silence about child molestation and abuse she experienced as a young girl, Carmen shares her authentic and honest story. This journey has led her to write her first non-fictional book, using her own story alongside the story of the Israelites in scripture who also suffered from the bondage of captivity to demonstrate a God who is invested in our freedom from every bondage – even in our mind and soul. She is a passionate advocate for broken and silent souls and has dedicated her life to helping restore people to their original "healthy" state - a person that is whole, free and that has the freedom to choose. This South African based author is also a mother of four and married to the love of her life, Wessel. If she is not writing she is cooking up a storm, painting, cycling, traveling, and enjoying every moment with her tribe in the beautiful Winelands of the Western Cape - with a glass of Pinotage, of course.

END NOTES

[1] "Motivational Quotations by Henry Ward Beecher." Quotes.thefamouspeople.com, quotes.thefamouspeople.com/henry-ward-beecher-1617.php. Accessed 19 July 2021.

[2] VILLANI, SUSAN. "Impact of Media on Children and Adolescents: A 10-Year Review of the Research." *Journal of the American Academy of Child & Adolescent Psychiatry*, vol. 40, no. 4, 2001, pp. 392–401., doi:10.1097/00004583-200104000-00007.

[3] Putnam, Dana E. "Initiation and Maintenance of Online Sexual Compulsivity: Implications for Assessment and Treatment." *CyberPsychology & Behavior*, vol. 3, no. 4, 2000, pp. 553–563., doi:10.1089/109493100420160.

[4] Goldstein, David S. "Adrenal Responses to Stress." *Cellular and Molecular Neurobiology*, vol. 30, no. 8, 2010, pp. 1433–1440., doi:10.1007/s10571-010-9606-9.

[5] Talmon, A., & Ginzburg, K. (2018). "Body self" in the shadow of childhood sexual abuse: The long-term implications of sexual abuse for male and female adult survivors. *Child Abuse & Neglect*, 76, 416–425. https://doi.org/10.1016/j.chiabu.2017.12.004

[6] "The Most Up-to-Date Pornography Statistics." *Covenant Eyes*, 25 Jan. 2021, www.covenanteyes.com/pornstats/.

[7] MobieG. "Adult Grooming." *MOBIEG*, MOBIEG, 27 Apr. 2021, www.mobieg.co.za/abuse/adult-grooming.

[8] "'You Grow up Hating Yourself': Why Child Abuse Survivors Keep – and Break – Their Silence." *The Guardian*, Guardian News and Media, 30 June 2019, www.theguardian.com/society/2019/jul/01/you-grow-up-hating-yourself-why-child-abuse-survivors-keep-and-break-their-silence.

[9] Kulii, B. T. (2001). Lorde, Audre. *African American Studies Center*. https://doi.org/10.1093/acref/9780195301731.013.46912

[10] "Sex Addiction Treatment Program Options." *PsychGuides.com*, www.psychguides.com/behavioral-disorders/sex-addiction/treatment/.

[11] "Sex Addiction Treatment Program Options." *PsychGuides.com*, www.psychguides.com/behavioral-disorders/sex-addiction/treatment/.

[12] "The Purpose of the Wilderness." *Key Truths*, 8 May 2021, www.keytruths.com/purpose-of-wilderness/.

[13] "Robert Frost Quotes." *BrainyQuote*, Xplore, ww.brainyquote.com/quotes/robert_frost_101249.

[14] Fretheim, Terence E. "Exodus: Interpretation: A Bible Commentary for Teaching and Preaching." *Alibris*, www.alibris.com/Exodus-Interpretation-A-Bible-Commentary-for-Teaching-and-Preaching-Terence-E-Fretheim/book/12198280.

[15] "American Society of Addiction Medicine." *ASAM Home Page*, www.asam.org/.

[16] Hall, Melissa, and Joshua Hall. The Long-Term Effects of Childhood Sexual Abuse: Counseling Implications. 2011.

[17] Seuss. *The Lorax*. Vision Australia Information Library Service, 1998.

[18] van der Kolk, Bessel. "The Body Keeps The Score." *Bessel Van Der Kolk, MD.*, www.besselvanderkolk.com/resources/the-body-keeps-the-score.

[19] Donohue, Maureen. "Post-Traumatic Stress Disorder (PTSD)." *Healthline*, Healthline Media, 12 Nov. 2019, www.healthline.com/health/post-traumatic-stress-disorder.

[20] Raypole, Crystal. "Dopamine Addiction: A Guide to Dopamine's Role in Addiction." *Healthline*, Healthline Media, 30 Apr. 2019, www.healthline.com/health/dopamine-addiction.

[21] Katehakis, Alexandra. "Childhood Trauma and Masturbation." *Psychology Today*, Sussex Publishers, www.psychologytoday.com/us/blog/sex-lies-trauma/201502/childhood-trauma-and-masturbation#:~:text=Often%20when%20a%20child%20undergoes%20abuse%20or%20trauma,from%20the%20betrayal.%20It%20is%20simply%20too%20overwhelming.

[22] "ADHD / ADD in Children Health Center: Parenting Help, Study Tips and More." *WebMD*, WebMD,

www.webmd.com/add-adhd/childhood-adhd/adhd-traumatic-childhood-stress).

[23] Robinson, Lawrence. "ADHD Medications." *HelpGuide.org*, 19 Apr. 2021, www.helpguide.org/articles/add-adhd/medication-for-attention-deficit-disorder-adhd.htm.

[24] "Vincent Van Gogh Quotes." *BrainyQuote*, Xplore, www.brainyquote.com/quotes/vincent_van_gogh_120866.

[25] Emery, David. "Did Mlk Say 'Our Lives Begin to End the Day We Become Silent'?" *Snopes.com*, https://www.snopes.com/fact-check/mlk-our-lives-begin-to-end/.

[26] *Cyberchaos*, groups.csail.mit.edu/mac/classes/6.805/articles/cda/cleaver-cyberchaos.html.

[27] "Inspirational Quotes at BrainyQuote." *BrainyQuote*, Xplore, www.brainyquote.com/.

[28] WilesCEO, Jeremy, et al. "How to Quit Porn... for Good." *Conquer Series*, 7 July 2021, conquerseries.com/15-mind-blowing-statistics-about-pornography-and-the-church/?ims=fb-091818b&utm_campaign=Porn%2BStats%2BFB%2Bad%2B-%2BSeptember%2B12%2C%2B2018&utm_source=Facebook&utm_medium=Facebook%2Bpost&utm_content=15%2BMind-Blowing%2BStatistics%2BAbout%2BPornography%2BAnd%2BThe%2BChurch.

[29] "Often It's the Deepest Pain Which Empowers You to Grow Into Your Highest Self Karen Salman Sohn Notsalmoncom: Meme on ME.ME." *Me.me*, me.me/i/often-its-the-deepest-pain-which-empowers-you-to-grow-5581202.

[30] Larry. "The Body Keeps the Score BY Bessel Van DER Kolk, Md." *MaleSurvivor*, Male Sexual Assault Support Forum | MaleSurvivor, 14 July 2020, forum.malesurvivor.org/threads/the-body-keeps-the-score-by-bessel-van-der-kolk-md.79164/page-3.

[31] About The Author Richard Turf. "Trauma Creates Change You Don't Choose." *The Minds Journal*, 26 Mar. 2021, themindsjournal.com/trauma-creates-change-you-dont-choose/.

[32] "The Purpose of the Wilderness." *Key Truths*, 21 Aug. 2021, www.keytruths.com/purpose-of-wilderness/.

[33] *Plutarch - What We Achieve Inwardly Will Change Outer Reality.*, www.englischezitate.de/zitat/plutarch/219801/.

[34] "Steve Jobs Quotes That Will Motivate You Forever." *YourSelf Quotes*, 24 Mar. 2021, www.yourselfquotes.com/steve-jobs-quotes/.

Made in the USA
Coppell, TX
25 October 2021